Alzheimer's Basic Caregiving
—an ABC Guide—

by Kathy Laurenhue, M.A.

Table of Contents

I. *The Condition*

Dementia is not normal aging
Dementia
Alzheimer's disease (AD)
Dementia with Lewy Bodies (DLB)
Multi-infarct Dementia (MID)
Mild Cognitive Impairment (MCI)

Early stage patterns
Middle stage patterns
Late stage patterns

Is it depression or dementia?
Pain
Assessing pain in the person with Alzheimer's
disease
How can we relieve pain in a person with Alzheimer's
disease?

II. *Communication and behavior*

Walking to clear the cobwebs
When mobility is not perceived as a positive
Guidelines for guiding people where you want them

Introduction

No one in our family ever suffered from insanity.
We've always enjoyed it.
—*Author Unknown*

For all the years that my mother had Alzheimer's disease (AD), I kept that plaque on my desk as a reminder that laughter is still the best medicine. I certainly wasn't always successful at keeping the demons of anger, guilt and sorrow at bay, but many years after my mother's death, I am still grateful for the gifts within the grief – the lemonade potential within the lemons, if you will.

This book is intended to be a highly practical and not entirely serious look at caring for people with Alzheimer's disease and related forms of dementia. AD is a terrible disease, but you won't survive the caregiving years if you don't keep your sense of humor, find the absurd within the awful, and awaken your curiosity over the odd ways the brain works.

I have been writing about Alzheimer's disease for 15 years now. I have developed hundreds of hours of curriculum for national long-term care companies throughout the U.S. and Australia, and for multi-media training companies and the National Alzheimer's Association. Yet one of the most rewarding things I've done was produce an international, award-winning newsletter for caregivers of people with Alzheimer's disease. This book and its companion, *Activities of Daily Living– an ADL Guide for Alzheimer's Caregivers*, are outgrowths of those 4-page monthly compositions.

What this book isn't: There are a great many ethical, financial and legal concerns that need to be addressed when someone has dementia. There are complex decisions to make about support services and who will provide care where. I am also a strong believer in meaningful occupation of people with dementia. In order to limit the length of this book, I have not addressed any of those topics here, but I have written about them in other formats, and may produce sequels. (See also Resources at the end of this book.)

One caution: People with Alzheimer's disease remain unique individuals. What works for one person may not work for another. What works today, may not work tomorrow and what didn't work yesterday may work today. There are no single right answers. Experiment. Try new approaches.

And **one disclaimer:** I am not a doctor or a nurse; nothing suggested on these pages is meant to substitute for medical supervision by qualified professionals. I've tried to provide accurate explanations and useful advice based on what is currently known about Alzheimer's disease, but new research and deeper understanding may invalidate what is stated here.

A few words about terminology

As the opening quote in the introduction might indicate, I don't believe in using words like "suffer" or "victim." There is tragedy in every human life; using a word like "victim" sets the other person apart and makes him an object of pity, as if we are not equal in our humanity. Such words also seem to be at odds with words like "hope" and "joy," which can still be a vital part of the lives of both caregiver and care receiver. In this book I want to share what I know about how we can connect with one another, no matter what our varying disabilities may be. What I learned from my mother and countless others with dementia is that everyone – *everyone* – has something to share if we are only open to their gifts.

On a more mundane note:

- I have tried to avoid saying "he or she" by simply alternating among the pronouns and hope that doesn't cause confusion.

- I have tended to use "dementia" and "Alzheimer's disease" (AD) interchangeably because AD is the most common form of dementia. I hope *that* doesn't cause confusion.

- Although it is sometimes awkward, I have steadfastly used the words "person with dementia" or "people with Alzheimer's disease," because the condition is always secondary to the individual. Sometimes I have just used "person" and hope that "with AD" is understood. At other times I've used "care receiver," but the goal is always to build a relationship in which the care flows both ways.

- "Caregiver" is usually used to indicate both family members and professionals. I recognize that the physical and emotional circumstances in which they are giving care are often quite different, but both families and professionals need the same understanding of the person who has dementia and what the condition has done to his brain. When I want to refer particularly to the relationship between family members, I often refer to the care receiver as a "loved one" even though it sounds like a funeral director speaking of the "dearly departed." Sometimes I find the English language woefully inadequate.

My basic tenets

Here are my immutable tenets for providing quality care to someone with Alzheimer's disease.

1. If you've met one person with Alzheimer's disease, you've met one person with Alzheimer's disease. People with AD (and related forms of dementia) may have a common condition, but they remain unique individuals, and the course of their disease is never entirely predictable.
2. Always treat the individual first, the condition second. It is more important to know the individual than the disease. (But knowing the disease is helpful, too.)
3. Fear is the most pervasive negative emotion in people with AD. It's up to us to make them feel safe and secure.
4. Pain is the most commonly undiagnosed condition in people with AD because they lose the ability to verbalize their discomfort. Look daily for nonverbal signs of pain, and check with a doctor about relieving it.
5. The person with Alzheimer's disease cannot control the progression of the disease in his body. Therefore it is up to us to adapt our care to his needs.
6. People with Alzheimer's disease retain the full range of human emotions and deserve to be treated as our equals – always with dignity, but rarely with solemnity. Sharing our sense of humor is a great equalizer.
7. People with dementia lose brain cells. They do not lose their desire to feel useful and valued. They still have gifts to contribute.
8. People with Alzheimer's disease always make sense to themselves. It's up to us to decipher their messages.

9. You will never win an argument with someone with Alzheimer's disease.

10. People with Alzheimer's disease always understand more than they can express, and they are usually excellent at "reading" nonverbal communication and sensing the emotional atmosphere.

11. People with dementia will always stay where they feel they belong. It's up to us to make them comfortable in their surroundings or to remove them to a more reassuring place.

12. The person with Alzheimer's disease is not deliberately trying to upset us. If he were, he would have a different diagnosis.

13. Always assume the person with AD is doing the best he can in any given situation.

14. When a person is willfully resistive, always look for the big five:
    a) fatigue
    b) frustration
    c) fear and confusion
    d) physiological discomfort
    e) environmental agitators.

15. People with Alzheimer's disease may not remember names, but they always know who loves them and whom they love.

  Alzheimer's basic caregiving

I.
The Condition

1 — Gaining a basic understanding of dementia

When I was young, I admired clever people.
Now that I am old, I admire kind people.
—*Abraham Heschel*

There is a wonderful Australian video on Alzheimer's disease (AD) called *You Must Remember This* in which the friends of a man with AD said they had a hard time recognizing it at first because they thought of him as "delightfully batty all the time." They realized that it was something more severe when he forgot an item that was completely out of character for him: the liquor for a party.

My father told me that my mother had gone to bed early one winter night. When she received a long-distance call from her brother in California, my father called from the living room for her to pick up the phone. He continued chatting with Uncle Richard for a little while, but when my mother didn't get on the line, he went to check on her. She was trying to listen through the control for the electric blanket. At the time I thought it was a funny story about waking up groggy, but it was a sign.

Woodrow Wirsig in his book, *I Love You, Too*, says his realization came when at breakfast his wife patted her hair and said, *I must get my shower cap done.*

Alone, none of these anecdotes would be alarming, but in each case they prompted remembrances of other incidents that indicated something was amiss.

Dementia is not normal aging

The ability of a normal aging adult to learn is lifelong. Older adults may be a little slower to learn new information or take longer to recall facts or take tests than their younger counterparts. However, an 80-year old brain has a lifetime of experiences and knowledge jammed inside; perhaps pulling up specific information takes longer simply because the 80-year old brain has much more to filter through than a 20-year old brain!

Older adults may also be a little less adept at remembering names and lists. Minor episodes of forgetfulness are to be expected at any age, especially when we are stressed. But memory loss characterized by Alzheimer's disease or any other form of dementia is *not* normal. If you are reading this book, chances are you are already a caregiver with an understanding of the particular form of dementia of your care receiver, but just so that we start out with a mutual understanding, allow me to give some basic information.

There are many books that provide detailed explanations about the parts of the brain affected by Alzheimer's disease. Others go into great detail about the dozens of variations of dementia. I prefer to avoid jargon and complicated terminology. I think it is more important for caregivers to understand the effects of Alzheimer's disease than the affected brain parts.

In recent years we have been learning more and more about preventive measures we can take against many of the diseases that are likely to be our cause of death, most of which are based on simple common sense:

- eat a balanced diet
- exercise regularly
- don't smoke
- get enough sleep
- surround yourself with loving friends
- keep your mind active
- have a cheerful attitude

  Alzheimer's basic caregiving

That's good advice for everyone, but the reality is we will still all die eventually from something. Genes, environment and lifestyle combine in ways we don't fully understand. In spite of our attempts to "live right" one of us may die of heart disease like our father and another of Alzheimer's disease like our mother. That's not an excuse to live recklessly, but it is an admonition not to blame the person who gets Alzheimer's disease for his condition.

Dementia is usually divided into two forms – reversible and irreversible. Irreversible dementias are the forms for which we currently know far too little about the causes and for which we have no cure, although we have *some* (limited) treatments.

That means – **and this is the single most important lesson of this book – the person with Alzheimer's disease cannot control the progression of the disease in his body.** His brain is being continuously assaulted and damaged; **therefore it is up to us to change how we care for him.**

Dementia =

- The loss of *multiple* intellectual functions (such as memory, communication, reasoning and judgment) severe enough to interfere with a person's daily functioning. Note: Dementia is more than just memory loss.

- **Not a disease itself but a symptom of many diseases,** generally categorized as reversible (curable) and irreversible (so far incurable).

- Dementia is **progressive**, meaning it will get worse over time, so that even reversible forms of dementia, if untreated, may eventually become irreversible.

- Common reversible dementias may be caused by such things as nutritional issues, thyroid conditions, a bad reaction to medication, depression, drugs or alcohol abuse, minor head injuries and certain brain tumors. (Not *all* drug and alcohol-induced dementias are reversible.)

- The three most common irreversible forms of dementia are Alzheimer's disease, Dementia with Lewy Bodies and multi-infarct dementia.

Because many forms of dementia *are* treatable, an early and accurate diagnosis is vital.

Alzheimer's disease (AD) =

- The **most common cause of dementia** (About 24 million people worldwide are believed to have it.)
- Named after Dr. Alois Alzheimer, a German doctor who found abnormal clumps (now called amyloid plaques) and bundles of fibers (now called neurofibrillary tangles) when he autopsied the brain of a patient in 1906. (We have since learned that some people who *don't* have dementia have these plaques and tangles in their brains when they die.)
- **Primary risk factor is age**, although one rare form of AD known as Early Onset can occur as early as the twenties.
- **Average life-expectancy after diagnosis is 8 – 10 years**, but some people live as long as 20 years.
- **Most common symptoms tend to be the loss of short-term memory, good judgment, visual-spatial skills, facility with numbers and language, and disorientation to time and place.** Over time, damage to the person's brain will also cause him to neglect personal safety, hygiene, and nutrition, which can lead to additional problems.

Dementia with Lewy Bodies (DLB)

Although not nearly as well known, Dementia with Lewy Bodies (sometimes called Diffuse Lewy Body Disease) is the second most common form of degenerative dementia in older adults. It may be less well known because there is confusion over whether it is a variant of Alzheimer's disease, Parkinson's disease or its own entity. It is named for the abnormal small, round structures (Lewy bodies, described in 1912 by Frederich Heinrich Lewy, M.D.) found in certain areas of the brain upon autopsy. These structures have long been associated with Parkinson's disease, but only about a third of people with Parkinson's disease develop dementia.

But if the origins of DLB are uncertain, the symptoms are fairly distinct:

- **Well-defined, vivid, visual hallucinations.** In DLB's early stage, the person may even acknowledge and describe the hallucinations. They may see a pet on a bed, for example. Visual hallucinations are often the first sign that distinguishes DLB. (People with Alzheimer's disease may have hallucinations later in the disease process.) Other types of hallucinations are less common but sometimes occur. These might be auditory ("hearing" sounds), olfactory (such as "smelling" food or paint) or tactile ("feeling" something that isn't there).

- **Mild problems with recent memory**, such as forgetting recent events.

- **Brief episodes of unexplained confusion and loss of abilities** like those associated with AD. (The person may not know where she is, may have trouble with speech, lose her way, lack judgment or insight, be inattentive or indecisive.)

- **Fluctuation in the occurrence of these episodes** from moment to moment, or week to week. For example, the person may converse normally one day and be mute, unable to speak the next day. Later, clarity may again return, just as unexpectedly. (This can occasionally occur in some other dementias, too.) This may cause others to think the person is "putting them on," or faking his symptoms.

- **Fluctuating problems with motor function** that are often found in Parkinson's disease, such as bent posture, shuffling gait, reduced arm-swing, limb stiffness, slowness of movement, and tremor. These motor function problems usually appear later in the disease process, but coupled with visual-spatial deficits (such as the ability to judge distances) and hallucinations, put them at high risk for falls.

Multi-infarct dementia (MID) =

- A form of dementia, also known as vascular dementia, **caused by a number of strokes in the brain.**

- These strokes **can affect some intellectual abilities, impair motor and walking skills, and cause an individual to experience hallucinations, delusions, or depression.**

- The **onset of MID is usually abrupt and often progresses in a stepwise fashion.** That means you are likely to notice sudden, significant changes, but after that a person may plateau for months or even years before another episode causes further deterioration.

- Individuals with MID are likely to have risk factors for strokes, such as high blood pressure, heart disease, or diabetes. Since risk can be lowered with lifestyle changes (better diet, more exercise, no smoking, etc.), **this form of dementia is somewhat preventable.**

Many people also have a combination of AD, MID and DLB.

Mild Cognitive Impairment (MCI)

In recent years many people have been diagnosed with Mild Cognitive Impairment after complaining of memory loss. MCI is abnormal and often leads to Alzheimer's disease over time, but unlike AD, MCI really is relatively mild as the name implies and refers only to memory loss. People with MCI do not have other losses like confusion, attention problems, and difficulty with language.

2 —Patterns of progression in Alzheimer's disease

I never forget a face,
But I'll make an exception in your case.
– Groucho Marx

Dr. Barry Reisberg of New York University has been studying Alzheimer's disease for decades. He gained notoriety early on by developing what he called a Global Deterioration Scale (GDS) which outlines the order in which people with Alzheimer's disease tend to lose specific skills. He came up with seven stages, although Stage 1 is basically any normal adult, and Stage 2 is any normally aging adult, so that concern only arises if people enter Stage 3. The later stages also have subsets: 7a, 7b, 7c and so on.

For a long time his work was somewhat controversial. Opponents felt that categorizing people with dementia – even into early, middle and late stage categories – was subjecting them to labels that limited expectations of them in the same way that expectations for a child who is labeled "learning disabled" in first grade has a hard time outgrowing teachers' lowered expectations during the ensuing years. The number one tenet to remember in this field is: **If you've met one person with Alzheimer's disease, you've met one person with Alzheimer's disease.** In other words, everyone with AD remains a unique individual and deserves to be treated as that individual, not as a "disease."

The National Alzheimer's Association now uses Reisberg's stages to help identify common patterns of progression, but always with this caveat: *[I]t is important to note that all stages are artificial benchmarks in a continuous process that can vary greatly from one person to another.*

I have long admired Dr. Reisberg's work, but I also agree with the caveat. In the video, *Inside Looking Out*, a woman with AD named Ruth is interviewed. She knows she is incompetent with numbers now and recognizes she needs help in that area, but she strongly objects to the idea that being unable to handle numbers makes her an incompetent person. Yet there is a strong tendency in many of us to discount people who have word-finding difficulties, for example. We make a huge mistake when we think that people who can no longer carry on easy conversations have lost their ability to understand what we say.

On the other hand, when a person who has been able to use the bathroom on his own begins to urinate in the garden, we need to be alert that he may be transitioning to a later stage and need a higher level of care. Or not. Perhaps he has a urinary tract infection that needs attention. Either way, changes alert us. If he is transitioning from Stage 6 to 7, chances are that we need to be on the lookout for other assistance he may need – with eating or bathing or communicating his wishes.

In the rest of this book I have avoided most mention of stages. The person is doing such-and-such because his brain is damaged by the disease, not necessarily because he is in Stage 4 or 6. But because I also want readers to have a sense of common patterns of progression in Alzheimer's disease, on the following pages are examples.

Early stage patterns

Using Dr. Barry Reisberg's Global Deterioration Scale, early stage dementia is equivalent to his Stages 3 and 4, middle stage is equivalent to his Stages 5 and 6, and late stage is equivalent to his Stage 7, but there is tremendous variation within each of those stages. For example:

In Stage 3, a person with AD may be unable to follow a map and consequently get lost driving to a new location. By Stage 4, he may still be able to find *familiar* locations, but he may misjudge the distance of an approaching car or be unable to interpret the meaning of a traffic signal, so that his impaired judgment makes him an unsafe driver.

In Stage 3, a person with AD may have gone from misplacing her glasses (Stage 2 = all of us!) to misplacing an object of real value, often wedding rings or other jewelry. By Stage 4, she may start to stash or hide objects for safekeeping, particularly if she is under the delusion that "people are stealing things." (See Chapter 10.) Sometimes, however, it may not be a matter of "hiding" as much as simply randomly "putting away" with no memory for where. People who want to try to preserve order usually find that labeling drawers and leaving notes works pretty well in these early stages.

We all lose our train of thought from time to time, particularly if we are under stress or there is a lot going on around us, but by Stage 3 people with AD will have word-finding difficulties, particularly for names, that go beyond the expected. By Stage 4, the give and take of normal conversations may be slowed, but if you allow the person with AD to set the pace and scope of the conversation, many can still do quite well.

Math deficits appear in Stage 3. As a family caregiver, you may notice this when your spouse asks you to take over the balancing of the checkbook, pay the cashier at the grocery store or figure the tip at a restaurant. You may also notice that your loved one is unsure of the day of the week or the date. By Stage 4, he misses the date by a week or more, and especially near transition months, may not remember the year. It is common for people in Stages 3 and 4 to have trouble telling time, especially when asked at any point that is not the hour or half hour. (Digital watches may make things easier, but I don't know of research proving that.)

Nevertheless, people in Stages 3 and 4 are "oriented to time and person," that is, they are living in the present, know who they are and recognize familiar faces, even if they can't always remember names. They may have forgotten some things in their personal past, but in Stage 3, they are usually able to recall at least one childhood teacher or friend. In Stage 4, the memories become more fragmented and fall out of chronological sequence, so that they may remember the schools they attended, but not their order. Their spouse – having heard the stories many times – is likely to recall more than they can.

In Stage 3, people can recall recent major events, but become flummoxed trying to answer detailed questions about these events. By Stage 4, they often can't recall even major events of the previous week or weekend, may not be able to recall what transpired the previous evening on their favorite televisions shows and are likely to have only vague knowledge of current events. They may read the newspaper but quickly forget what they've read.

People who are still working are likely to lose their jobs at this point, but if you and your spouse are retired, you are more likely to notice deficits in household chores. Your wife is no longer able to follow a recipe and begins to avoid cooking. She no longer wants to do the grocery shopping because the massive aisles of products and the decisions to be made are too confusing. Your husband doesn't remember how to mow the lawn or use his power tools and may have an accident or destroy equipment trying. However, jobs that require repetitive actions may still be able to be done with ease: hanging clothes on a line (as opposed to operating the controls on a dryer), ironing, sanding wood, (sometimes) painting.

  Alzheimer's basic caregiving

Social events may begin to be avoided because they are too confusing. Your loved one may have forgotten the rules to playing cards or bingo, or may no longer be able to add up his golf score. She may make excuses to avoid going to church or synagogue where she is expected to greet and recognize people whom she has forgotten. You will notice a withdrawal from situations perceived as intimidating, but the reasons given are likely to be a "cover up": *I've lost interest* or *I don't feel like it today.* If you press her, she may become angry. This is where the Alzheimer's Association tends to identify a personality change, but I disagree. It's a coping mechanism; if I'm afraid I can't do something or – even more frightening – afraid that I am losing my mind, it's quite logical to do my best to pretend I don't *want* to do that thing and hope you won't notice my deficit.

When one spouse has AD, this early stage is often a strain on marriages because the way a couple has done things for 50 years suddenly isn't working anymore. Change is hard, especially if the person with dementia is perceived as "just being stubborn," or "just trying to irritate me." A person with AD may indeed be willfully resistant to a request, but the resistance is based on the person's underlying fear or confusion or simple fatigue (concentrating takes too much energy). The person is not deliberately trying to upset his or her spouse or other family caregiver. This situation tends to be aggravated by the fact that the well family member doesn't *want* to believe something serious is wrong.

Middle stage patterns

People with early stage dementia can usually still live alone with some assistance, especially if they have a spouse or adult child to help "fill in the gaps." Assistive devices can also help.

By the middle stage or according to Reisberg's GDS, Stage 5, people with AD are no longer capable of living safely on their own, although again, many people will continue to live at home under the careful supervision of a spouse, adult child or other caregiver. Others will move to an assisted living community or nursing home at this point.

Those who are living in a residential care community often look like visitors. They may be dressed up as if they are going out: men in suits or natty sports clothes with keys and wallets in their pockets; women in dresses, hose, make-up, jewelry and carrying purses. What's more, they often believe they *are* visitors – why else would they be carrying their purses? If you come in as a real visitor, you may find that you can talk with a person in Stage 5 for several minutes without realizing she has dementia, especially if she is having a good day.

People in Stage 5 are dressed up because they believe they still have responsibilities (places to go and people to see), but their perceptions of their responsibilities are based on *misperceptions,* and they don't welcome your interference. They still have volition; they can form a thought, plan an action and follow-through. (Although some people may lose their train of thought along the way, lose the goal, and are perceived by others as purposeless wanderers.) Typically, they are living in (or float in and out of) a past reality so that a woman may believe she must be at home when her children return from school. Look for agitation at what would have been normal transition times in their daily routines, such as mid- to late afternoon. If you dare to suggest her children are long grown, her reaction is likely to be panic that you don't believe her. (This topic is discussed further in Chapter 8.)

When you consider that they are often living at least part-time in a past reality, it is not surprising that people in the middle stage have increasing difficulty with time and dates. Indeed, time begins to lose its meaning. *I'll be back in 10 minutes,* is not something they may be able to differentiate from 10 hours. They may have no idea what season it is without daily reminders: *Good morning, George! Time to get up; it's a beautiful spring morning.*

In Stage 5, math, number and language deficits tend to grow more pronounced. People may not remember their address or phone. They may not be able to retain the names of three items on a grocery list or tell you a watch is a watch. But many people at this stage are aware of their growing deficits and anxious about them. They often try to hang onto every bit of independence they can, so that if you are a female caregiver and you tell a man with AD that it is time for him to get dressed, he is likely to say, *Who died and made you boss?*

However, most of today's older men were raised with courtly manners, and years of "honey-do" lists from their wives and mothers. If, instead of giving an order, you can preface your request with a phrase like, *Could you please help me with this?* you are likely to be more successful.

Both their manners and their deeply ingrained tendency to be helpful make people in this stage natural hosts and greeters, so tap into this at social events. Station them at the door to welcome others or ask them to pass out drinks or desserts. Precisely because they want to hang onto their remaining strengths, they appreciate opportunities to be helpful. In residential or day care settings they will often "parent" people in Stage 6 by helping with activities or grooming tasks such as brushing someone's hair. Cameron Camp, Ph.D., director of the Myers Research Institute, has had success involving people in Stages 5 and 6 in a comedy club. Some people can still tell their own jokes, but Cameron provides others in large print on strips of paper that can be drawn from a hat and read. People who don't want to be jokesters are given other tasks – greeter, lemonade distributor, and audience members.

People in Stage 5 are usually able to go the bathroom on their own and eat on their own. They may be able to help with basic food preparation such as chopping vegetables, snapping beans, or stirring the cake batter, but they usually cannot be counted on to use a stove safely or follow a recipe without supervision. They tend to lose visual-spatial abilities so that setting a table or loading a dishwasher may be too challenging. They can still handle most grooming tasks, but some need their choices simplified – their clothes laid out in the order for putting them on, toothpaste put on their toothbrush and distractions such as cologne, lotions and hair spray removed from their line of vision. (This is definitely needed by Stage 6.)

Stage 5 is also when individual strengths are likely to begin showing up. Someone who was an accountant may not have the math deficits typical of this stage. A person who always did crossword puzzles and other word games may still be better than her peers at them. People who play a musical instrument may make some mistakes, but retain the basic skill until very late in the disease process.

There are also physical changes that tend to take place in Stage 5 as damage in the brain spreads to the hypothalamus – the part of the brain that controls body temperature and sleep. Difficulty sleeping or sleeping for an hour or two and then getting up and walking around are common in Stage 5 (and/or 6) and understandably upsetting to family caregivers who need their rest. People in Stage 5 also have a tendency to be colder than the rest of us, and as we discuss in Chapter 7, nighttime restlessness and the tendency to be cold are sometimes related.

The primary motivation of people in Stage 6 is comfort. In terms of dress, people in Stage 6 are seldom interested in keeping up appearances. If you've ever come home from a night of partying or from work after a long day of "looking professional" and the first thing you do is take off your jewelry, your belt and your shoes, you have an idea of how a person in Stage 6 is likely to react to being "gussied up." Comfort for a person in Stage 6 can also extend to removing eyeglasses, dentures and hearing aides, and that requires vigilance. I know of one nursing home resident who, as she finished toileting, scratched her ear, felt the hearing aid, took it off and looked at it, and before anyone realized what was happening, flushed it down the toilet. When questioned about what she had done, she said, *I threw that turd away.* Many share the sentiment.

Pay attention to the fact that seeking comfort may be based on experiencing real discomfort. Glasses may be dirty or the prescription may no longer be appropriate. Dentures may not fit well anymore or they may have food particles caught beneath them. Hearing aids may be hard for the person to adjust or may not seem to help. Pay attention to the message behind the behavior because by this time, a person's ability to verbally express the cause of his discomfort is long gone.

If you haven't done so before, Stage 6 is the time to simplify. People in Stage 6 often resist changing clothes, probably for a number of logical reasons:

- Their ability to dress themselves independently has disappeared, and left to their own devices, they may put pants on backwards, shoes on the wrong feet or underwear over pants.

- They may have some awareness of their difficulties; therefore, once they are dressed, they see no reason to change clothes, and may find even the thought exhausting.
- They may also find the process literally painful as physical changes make them less flexible or chronic conditions such as arthritis intensify.
- They may find the ordinary clothes they wore in the past challenging. Stage 6 is when clothes that pull on, pull over, slip on, fit loosely, feel soft, zip rather than button and tighten with Velcro rather than shoestrings, are all appropriate.

By Stage 6, people have usually given up their sense of responsibility, so that you no longer have to talk them out of going to work or getting home to make supper for their children. Some people in this stage – having forgotten what they have forgotten – are fairly content and easily pleased by simple kindness or a little attention. Others seem to wake each day feeling like strangers in a strange land. They often do not know where they are and have a fear of being alone. If you ask someone in Stage 6 who is living in an assisted living residence where she is, her answer is likely to be the most logical place she can come up with based on a past reality or the size of the place. She may think she is in a college dormitory, a hotel, on a cruise, or any number of other places in a city where she once lived. Often her comfort with her surroundings is somewhat precarious, based on being in view of friendly faces or someone she knows. Therefore, she may follow you everywhere you go (called "shadowing") and may ask questions like, *Where should I be?* or *What should I do?* Some people will sit quietly for hours as long as a person they feel safe with is present. Others are looking for things to occupy them. They can still successfully participate in activities requiring repetitive actions (sweeping, folding napkins, wiping counters),

  Alzheimer's basic caregiving

simple sorting (poker chips by color, screws from bolts) or rote memory (washing dishes, singing songs) to name just a few examples.

This is a time when language abilities diminish significantly and when recent memory constantly disappears so that for the person in Stage 6 yesterday might never have happened. However, feelings remain strong. A person may not remember what happened at lunch to upset her, but the feelings of being upset may linger through the afternoon unless something pleasant happens to counteract it.

People in Stage 6 tend to need significant assistance with all their dressing and grooming tasks including toileting. They may begin to be incontinent of bladder and bowel. If they didn't begin to have a disruption of their sleep/wake cycle in Stage 5, they may have it now, but others begin to need more sleep, including more daytime naps.

They usually still respond to their own name ("Mary" – not "Mother" or "Mrs. Jones") but they no longer recognize themselves in the mirror, probably because they are living in a past reality now more or less full-time; they may believe they are young mothers or even school children, so the old woman in the mirror is not someone they know. For this same reason – the fact that they imagine themselves much younger – they often do not know the names of many of the people who are close to them (or do not associate our aging faces with the names), although they will respond to familiar faces and they always know who loves them and whom they love.

Late stage patterns

In the late stage of Alzheimer's disease – Reisberg's Stage 7 – people eventually become totally dependent. They need assistance with all their ADLs (activities of daily living such as dressing, bathing, grooming), become incontinent of both bladder and bowel, and often need assistance with eating (although many can manage finger foods for quite a long while). They often speak only a few coherent words and sometimes none at all, although they still tend to understand much more than they can express, and occasionally pop out with a whole sentence that surprises everyone.

Their bodies look abnormal. Their tendency to list to one side and to lose their balance (which usually begins in Stage 6) becomes more exaggerated. Their faces often look blank, and they may seem to be lost in thought. It becomes more difficult to gain and hold their attention. Both their increasing vision problems and their loss of propriaception (knowing where their body is in space) tend to make them unsure of their footing so that they go about with a downward gaze, giving them a bellybutton view of the world. They lose the ability to stay balanced while standing still, and it becomes increasingly difficult for them to step sideways, turn around, or back up. Once they have attained forward motion, they may be able to keep going for awhile, but keeping them from falling and bumping into things is a major problem. Because their stamina decreases, they need way stations – benches or other resting places – but these can also become obstacles in their paths. They may hang onto tables or push a chair along for balance, and then bruise themselves on that same aid. People in this stage look to their environment for cues, but principally they look at floors. Because they lose their 3-D vision, they see darkness as depth and a dark carpet or checkerboard tile floor as holes, making walking even trickier. Sunlight streaming into a room may create confusing patterns on a carpet; sunlight through blinds may create step-like shadows. At the same time, stairs without color contrasting strips on the edges blend together as a single surface. All of this, of course, can lead easily to falls and bruises and broken bones.

My colleague Roseann Kasayka, Ph.D., has noted that scans which show brain wave activity in meditating monks and people in late stage Alzheimer's disease are remarkably similar. It may be possible that people with late stage AD are actually in a peaceful meditative state. It's an intriguing thought worth further pursuit.

On the other hand, it's still possible to engage a person who is in Stage 7. Their eyes tend to be drawn to things that move or sparkle or light up and to strong contrasts like bulls' eyes. They still react to sounds of nature and music and to touch – a gentle hand massage or the feel of satin, fur or flannel, for example. They may still enjoy fiddle objects, repetitive motion tasks and walking hand in hand or even waltzing down the hallway. (People unsteady on their feet can often do better moving to the rhythm of a slow dance.) Most will enjoy laughing and smiling nearly until their dying day.

Stage 7 is the last phase of Alzheimer's disease. Eventually most people become bed-ridden as they lose the ability to walk; they need to be fed by hand until swallowing problems signal that the body is shutting down. Many will acquire pneumonia from aspirating food, but most can be helped to a peaceful death if they are surrounded by a caring community. In my experience, various hospice organizations are superb in making sure this happens. Others have developed Alzheimer's-specific palliative care programs. (See Resources.)

3—Dementia, depression and pain

Just because you're miserable
doesn't mean you can't enjoy your life.
—Annette Goodheart, Ph.D.

The focus of this chapter is "heavy" but that doesn't mean that facing up to what needs to be addressed leaves out all opportunity for good humor. Indeed, finding things to laugh about or be cheerful about are two of the best antidotes to pain and depression, and dementia is no barrier to enjoyment. Or as Mark Twain once said, *Whatever a man's age, he can reduce it several years by putting a bright-colored flower in his buttonhole.*

Dementia, depression and pain are three strands of a tightly woven rope making it difficult to separate one from the other.

- People who have a diagnosis of Alzheimer's disease often go through a period of depression, which is not surprising, given that it is a terminal illness.

- But other people with potentially reversible dementia may be depressed because they know something is terribly wrong and are afraid to learn exactly what it is. They may withdraw from friendships and normal activities, which further isolates them and may make both their depression and their dementia worse, particularly if they aren't eating well. (Malnutrition can also contribute to signs of dementia.)

- On the other hand, people may be depressed due to chronic pain from arthritis or some other condition. If they also have dementia, they may not know how to take medications to relieve that pain or how to express that pain to others.

- Other people with depression may develop aches and pains from their inactivity.

Are you confused yet? Perhaps you can see why an accurate diagnosis is vital to treatment. Reversible dementia, by definition, is treatable. We also have an increasing number of approved drugs for Alzheimer's disease, and we know much more than we once did about how to meet the daily emotional needs of people with AD and related forms of dementia. Pain and depression are also treatable if they are recognized. The difficulty can be treating the right symptom in the right way.

Is it depression or dementia?

Many older people who have experienced a traumatic loss such as the death of a spouse or a move from their home of 50 years, will exhibit signs of forgetfulness or disorientation that are upsetting to them – and to their families. Often this is aggravated by poor nutrition and fatigue. The widow who has lovingly cooked for her husband throughout their marriage often finds she doesn't have much interest in eating now that he has died. The widower who slept next to his wife for most of his life, may find it difficult to fall asleep without the heat and smell and touch of her beside him. Winifred Gallagher in her book *The Power of Place* describes grief as not just a psychological sense of loss, but a multi-sensory physiological loss as well. It should also be noted that most older adults have experienced *multiple* losses, such as the Four Ds:

- **Deaths** of a number of relatives and friends.
- **Deterioration** in their own health which may result in greater isolation from remaining friends and pleasures. Perhaps they can no longer drive or choose not to drive to evening events because of deteriorating vision. Perhaps a hearing impairment keeps them from going

out to eat because noisy restaurants make it hard for them to hear conversation. Perhaps going to social or educational events takes too much of their now limited energy. The list goes on.

- **Distance** from family and long-time friends. Few older adults live close to all their children, grandchildren and siblings because families have scattered in recent decades. Chances are also good that the person you have known and cherished since grade school no longer lives in the neighborhood.

- **Diminished** space. Many people willingly downsize when their children leave home, and are happy to see their children's pleasure in the furniture or china they pass on to them, but that doesn't mean they don't mourn – at least temporarily – the home and possessions they have given up.

We would not be human if these losses didn't sadden us. But not all sadness leads to clinical depression and accompanying memory loss. How can you tell if someone's memory problems are a sign of Alzheimer's disease or depression? It is an oversimplification, but one way is to ask the person a question. The person with Alzheimer's disease, at least in the early stages, tends to want to conceal her memory loss, so she will answer the question as well as she can, and if you tell her she is wrong, she will make up an excuse about why she missed it. She becomes so adept at this that she can often conceal her losses even from family members for quite awhile. She may rely heavily on notes and calendars and sometimes post-its stuck in odd places to keep up the appearance that all is well. Because the onset of Alzheimer's disease is usually slow, it sometimes goes unnoticed by outsiders for years.

The person whose memory loss is connected to depression tends to be much more apathetic. She may ignore the question you ask, say immediately, *I don't know,* without thinking, or say she isn't interested in "playing your games." She may complain of not only her loss of memory but lots of other problems as well. Her family is acutely aware of her condition – whose beginning can often be tied to a specific event, such as the death of a spouse or an illness – because she reminds them regularly. Her apathy for doing things may extend to household tasks and her personal appearance, and her deterioration often proceeds rapidly.

At the same time, people with Alzheimer's disease may also be depressed or exhibit signs of anxiety, tearfulness and agitation (all signs of depression), particularly in the early to middle stages of the disease when their awareness of their losses is greatest. These symptoms may increase in the afternoon as they begin to tire from other events of the day.

A majority of people who are depressed – whether or not it is related to Alzheimer's disease – can usually be helped by anti-depressants and counseling or participation in a support group. Depression is a serious condition that requires a qualified doctor's care, particularly because it increases the risk for suicide. The highest rate of suicide in the U.S. is among adults 70 and older. Peter Birkett, M.D., in his book, *Psychiatry in the Nursing Home,* says that this is not the time (as with anti-psychotics) "to go low and go slow." Rather, the dosage needs to be high enough to be effective, a factor which can be determined scientifically by your physician.

All of the medications taken by any older adult should be monitored and re-evaluated periodically by a physician. This is especially important in people with Alzheimer's disease or a related form of dementia, because the brain's deterioration may make certain medications ineffective or unnecessary over time. Some medications have a potential side effect of lowering our mood, so sometimes stopping one medication can make anti-depressants superfluous. Virginia Morris in her book, *How to Care for Aging Parents*, quotes one woman whose mother was atypically apathetic about a granddaughter's upcoming wedding. When her mother next saw her doctor, he re-evaluated her medications and greatly reduced the dosage of a blood pressure medication she had been taking for 18 years. Her mother's spirits returned, and she was the life of the (wedding) party.

It should also be noted, however, that as caregivers we can have a profound effect on people with dementia. They need loving gestures, kind words, hugs and activities that distract and engage them. They need to see that they still have a role in life and are still valued. We can often improve the spirits of others by simply involving them in an activity they enjoy.

We also need to know that sometimes our best intentions misfire. *A little boy with a small scratch on his finger sadly sought his mother. When he found her, she was pre-occupied and unconcerned. She said, "Well, what can I do about it?" The little boy replied, "You could say, 'Ouch'."* On the one hand, people with Alzheimer's disease want the acknowledgement that what they have is a serious and awful condition. When we make light of their disability by saying things like, *Oh, don't worry. I forget lots of things, too,* Larry Rose says it is like saying, *Other than that, Mrs. Lincoln, how did you like the play?* If someone tells you he has Alzheimer's disease, we should have the decency to say, *Ouch,* and acknowledge that is a rough card to be dealt.

On the other hand, one reason many people try to hide their disabilities with Alzheimer's disease is that they don't want our pity or sympathy. They want to continue to be accepted as human beings with the full range of human emotions, skills they can still use, and gifts they can still contribute. They want to be treated as normally as possible, and they want us to keep laughing and crying with them in ways that we always have. One of the reasons that the Best Friends series of books on Alzheimer's disease written by Virginia Bell and David Troxel struck a chord with so many people is that it reduced what was for many a scary, mysterious disease to a simple matter of caring just as we would for a good friend.

Pain

When people with dementia are a pain in the neck, it's often because they have a pain in their leg – or hand or back or tummy.

Consultant Mary Lucero, my first mentor in the field of dementia caregiving, often tells this (paraphrased) story:

One day when the family of a man in a nursing home came to visit, he accosted them upon their arrival saying they needed to get him to a hospital right away because "I've been shot by wild Indians with bows and arrows!" To suggest that his family didn't believe him was putting it mildly. Indeed, they chastised him for creating a scene and told him his story was preposterous. Now the one thing that you can be sure will never calm someone with Alzheimer's disease is telling him you don't believe him. So again the man cried out, "Help me! I've been shot by wild Indians with bows and arrows!" Fortunately, a nurse happened along and since she was wearing her sensible shoes that day, she asked him the logical question: "Mr. Jones, where does it hurt?" because anyone knows that if you have been shot with bows and arrows, you are likely to be in pain – a message that hadn't penetrated the skulls of the man's family who (like most of us would be) were busy being embarrassed for their loved one. Mr. Jones was able to point to his shoulder, which the nurse promptly

examined, and indeed his bursitis was badly inflamed. She treated the bursitis and the pain, and Mr. Jones went on to enjoy a quiet visit with his family.

The story illustrates a number of common problems in recognizing pain in people with dementia:

- For reasons that are still poorly understood, most people with Alzheimer's disease, particularly as their condition progresses, cannot or do not express their discomfort with simple words: *My shoulder hurts.*

- They do express their pain through their behavior which is frequently anxious or agitated. (See more detail below.)

- In the later stages of Alzheimer's disease, hallucinations and delusions are relatively common. Hallucinations and delusions that are frightening or otherwise indicate discomfort are often an expression of physical pain that needs to be treated.

- The real message behind the behavior, hallucination or delusion is usually missed, which means that pain is severely under-treated in people with Alzheimer's disease.

Prevalence of Pain

Here are a few terrible statistics on pain:

- Pain is the most common chief complaint presented to primary care physicians.

- It has been estimated that chronic pain is the third largest health problem in the United States.

- Physicians and researchers have estimated that 70 - 85 percent of nursing home residents have significant pain.

- In a chart review of 60 non-verbal patients on an Alzheimer's unit, nurse Lynn Marzinski found that

26 had chronic conditions which could potentially have been painful, but only three received scheduled analgesics.

- It has been noted that nurses chart less than 50 percent of what patients describe, and that pain is most often assessed by patients' verbal expressions of discomfort.
- Nurses attribute less intense pain when the patient has no signs of pathology and when duration is chronic. (There is a natural tendency in most of us to ignore the chronic complainer over time.)
- Both professional nurses and family caregivers often look at chronic pain as psychological rather than physiological in origin.
- Anecdotal hospice research indicates that 80% of Alzheimer's patients die with unresolved pain issues.

Some won't mention it.

In spite of this widespread prevalence, part of the reason pain is under-assessed and under-treated is that older adults often fail to report pain. The reasons include:

- They believe it is a natural result of aging that simply must be endured.
- Their cultural values may call for stoicism; they believe it's not acceptable to show pain.
- They fear that if they complain they may lose their autonomy through hospitalization or institutionalization.
- They fear that if they complain they may be subjected to uncomfortable tests or expensive procedures they can ill afford.
- Their terminology is different. They say "no" when asked if they're in pain, and "yes" when asked if they have discomfort, soreness, aches or hurts.
- Drug interactions or side effects alter their perception of pain or the ability to report it.

- As we've already noted, dementia has robbed them of the vocabulary they need to describe their discomfort.

The consequences of failing to treat pain

Untreated pain:

- Increases stress
- Delays healing; inhibits the immune system
- Interferes with sleep
- Tends to reduce appetites and lower the chance for adequate nutritional intake
- Compromises mobility and puts people at increased risk for falls
- Can raise heart rates and blood pressure and exacerbate other medical conditions
- Is a primary contributor to depression
- Causes unnecessary suffering

This is only a partial list, but it should be obvious that pain is neither normal nor benign. Personally, I believe one reason untreated pain is highly prevalent and vastly under-treated in people with Alzheimer's disease is that people miss the message. They see the agitation caused by the pain and prescribe an anti-anxiety medication without treating the underlying cause. **My educated guess is that huge numbers of the behaviors that are so upsetting to family and professional caregivers would disappear if people were given regular treatment for the pain they do not verbalize.** But whether or not behavior changes, perhaps the greatest tragedy related to our treatment of Alzheimer's disease is the needless suffering caused by our failure to treat physical discomfort.

Assessing pain in the person with Alzheimer's disease

Aside from paying attention to described hallucinations and anxious behavior, there are many signs of pain that are observable. For example:

1. Noisy breathing
   - Breathing is labored, difficult
   - Respirations sound loud, harsh or gasping
   - Episodic bursts of rapid breaths or hyperventilation

2. Negative vocalization
   - Hushed low sounds such as constant guttural muttering
   - Repeating words in a mournful tone
   - Moans, groans, direct expressions of pain
   - Speech with a disapproving quality
   - General irritability

3. Facial expressions
   - Clenched jaw
   - Troubled or distorted face – looking hurt, worried, lonely, fearful, distressed, alarmed, pleading
   - Frowning – wrinkled brow, down-turned mouth, scowling
   - Lackluster eyes, glazed eyes, dilated pupils, tears, crying, tightly closed or widely opened eyes
   - Tightly closed or widely opened mouth

4. Body position/language
   - Clenched fists or wringing hands
   - Knees pulled up tightly into abdomen
   - Tension in extremities, strained and inflexible position
   - Rocking

- Guarding or appearing to protect painful area, such as keeping an arm in front of one's stomach
- Hunched shoulders

5. Fidgeting, pacing
  - Restless, impatient motion, increased hand/finger movements
  - Squirming, jittery, inability to keep still
  - Appearance of trying to escape area of hurt (which may be the reason for walking about)
  - Altered gait, posture
  - Forceful touching, tugging or rubbing of body parts

6. Aggression
  - Threatening gestures
  - Hostility
  - Striking out
  - Increased volume of voice

7. Change in daily activities, habits
  - Insomnia or other sleep disturbances
  - Loss of appetite, weight loss
  - Constipation or incontinence
  - Decreased ability to concentrate
  - Withdrawal from activities or relationships

Other experts suggest that it is a *change* in behavior that tends to be significant. There are some people who, when they are not engaged in an activity, will drone all day long. It seems to be a self-comforting technique. If that person suddenly stops droning, it may be a sign of infection or other condition causing discomfort. The opposite – someone who says nothing from morning to night and suddenly starts moaning – should also be viewed as a potential cause for concern. A person who has been easy-going and is suddenly restless needs evaluation. Let change alert you.

How can we relieve pain in a person with Alzheimer's disease?

Author and lecturer Leo Buscaglia often tells the story of a four-year old boy whose next door neighbor was an elderly gentleman whose wife had recently died. Upon seeing the man cry, the little boy went into the old gentleman's yard, climbed onto his lap, and just sat there. When his mother asked what he had said to the neighbor, the little boy said: *Nothing, I just helped him cry.* It's something we all can do.

A great deal of the care that is given to anyone with a chronic illness is palliative, that is, comfort care. We cannot cure people with dementia, but we can prevent negative reactions and increase their contentment through sensitivity to what they are telling us non-verbally.

As we all know, pain can sometimes be alleviated simply by changing the environment. If you ever have had a headache in traffic, shopping crowds or at a children's birthday party, you know how environment contributes to pain.

Sometimes it's a matter of changing the person's position or adjusting padding and pillows to alleviate a crick in the neck or a cramped arm. Adaptive devices exist to fit almost every need these days. Walking with a person who has been sitting too long can also relieve painful joints for some people. Moderate exercise is a powerful antidote to muscle stiffness.

Many people are uncomfortable simply because they are too hot or too cold and need a sweater or a change in clothing. Sometimes they can benefit from localized heat or cold compresses or simply elevating feet that have swollen. Many solutions are simple.

Diet may also play a role. Food is used by many of us to provide comfort – we bring a casserole to a funeral and

Alzheimer's basic caregiving

eat a chocolate bar when we're under stress. Mealtimes often become the high point of the day for someone who has few other pleasures, and as caregivers, we are tempted to indulge every whim. The side effects can be more pain in the form of heartburn (*I can't believe I ate the whole thing!*) or constipation. But diet can also be used to *relieve* pain by doing your best to help the person eat nutritionally.

Distraction, as briefly mentioned, is also often an effective pain reliever. Tension tends to tighten muscles and increase pain. If we can get someone to relax and laugh or sing with us, tension – and often pain – eases.

The most common form of pain relief, however, is medicine. When we have a headache, we take an analgesic – aspirin, ibuprofen (Advil, Motrin), acetaminophen (Tylenol) or, in severe cases, something stronger. If you suspect pain is the cause of certain behaviors, check with the person's doctor to see if there is any reason *not* to administer a pain reliever. Chronic conditions, such as arthritis, are often treated in institutional settings by dispensing medications on a PRN basis, which means, as needed, based on the person's request. For people with dementia, a fixed schedule under a doctor's supervision (allowing for experimentation in time, frequency and dosage) is usually more appropriate.

And sometimes it's not what we think

But before you attribute every action in a person with dementia to an expression of pain, it's important to note that much is still unknown, and many actions have different origins. The person who is agitated by watching disturbing images on the evening news can often be "cured" by simply turning off the TV and engaging him in a more enjoyable activity. Some things that *should* cause pain – or that do in younger people – affect older people differently. Some physicians have noted that heart attacks, peptic ulcer disease, appendicitis and pneumonia may cause only mild discomfort. Medicine is still in its infancy in understanding older adults!

II.
Communication
and Behavior

4 —Communication 101: It's a two-way affair

*The real art of conversation is not only to say
the right thing in the right place,
but to leave unsaid the wrong thing at the tempting moment.*
—Lady Dorothy Nevill

Communication is about messages, not just words. We express ourselves more honestly and eloquently with our actions, faces, body language and tone of voice than with what we actually say. (In fact, widely quoted studies by Albert Mehrabian, Ph.D., suggest 93% of our communication comes from those sources.) If you ask, *How are you?* nearly all of us will say, *Fine, thank you.* However, if you ask someone, and he says, *FINE!* in a tense or angry tone, with clenched jaw and fists, you know he is using the universal acronym for FINE: Frustrated, Insecure, Neurotic and Exhausted. Treat him especially gently.

And if you are the one with the clenched fists and jaw, no one with Alzheimer's disease will hear your words because your body language speaks much louder. Chances are fairly good that you violated the #1 rule for communicating with a person with AD, which is, *NEVER argue.* As any Alzheimer's expert in the country will tell you, **no one has ever won an argument with someone with Alzheimer's disease**. If like Helen Keller, you do not want the peace which passeth understanding, but the understanding which bringeth peace, read on.

Basic courtesy

Effective communication with anyone begins with common courtesy, and common courtesy begins with treating the person with Alzheimer's disease as your equal. Many books have been written about power plays, particularly in business. If you want to show your power over another person, you will put a barrier, such as a desk, between you and the person you are talking with. Or you will sit behind the desk while the person stands in front of it, and continue with your work, arranging papers or writing as the person talks. Or you will create barriers with your body by folding your arms across your chest and raising a skeptical eyebrow when he talks. The essential message I get from those techniques is that power players are rude.

To communicate effectively with people with Alzheimer's disease, begin by showing courteous interest:

- Stop whatever you are doing and give the person your undivided attention.
- Put your body at the same level or slightly below hers. If the person is in a wheelchair, sit down, too, or crouch beside her.
- Stand or sit close to the person with no barriers between you.
- Make eye contact, and, if appropriate, body contact by holding her hand or occasionally touching his arm.
- Call the person by his preferred name. While this is a courteous thing to do in any circumstance, it is particularly important when talking with people with Alzheimer's disease because it helps them to understand that you are talking to them specifically and that they need to "tune in." Even then, it may be necessary for you to call them by name three times or more before they make eye contact and focus on you.
- Keep your body language warm, open and friendly and your attitude optimistic. When we believe a conversation will go well, that has a powerful effect on actual outcomes.

You will also communicate more effectively when you remember to use "please" and "thank you," and other terms of appreciation and praise. We often get so used to giving orders to the person with AD that we forget to acknowledge their helpfulness.

Common courtesy also means that we never scold, make fun of or belittle a person with Alzheimer's disease. When someone has made a mess, set your schedule back, or created more work for you, it can be hard to keep your temper in check. Sarcasm is second nature for some people and hard to control. Many people believe that belittling someone for her mistakes will keep her from repeating them, when all it really does is make her afraid of you or uncomfortable in your presence.

On the other hand, don't spend your days walking on eggs. Most people with Alzheimer's disease enjoy good-natured bantering, joking, and kidding around. If you offend someone in the process, apologize sincerely, and refrain from doing it again, but the occasions when that is necessary are likely to be rare. Most people with AD want to be treated as normally as possible, and laughing together is a terrific "normal" activity.

Many people think that diminished vocabulary in people with AD equates to diminished understanding. Never underestimate what people with Alzheimer's disease understand, and never say anything in their presence that you wouldn't want them to understand. Common courtesy demands that you never speak to a third person as if the person with AD is not there. Always include them in conversations. For example, if you are an aide caring for Mrs. Jones, and while you are walking down the hall with her, Mrs. Jones' daughter arrives and asks you, *Did my mother have a good day?* a courteous response would be, *Well, how would you rate your day, Mrs. Jones? You enjoyed the gardening class, didn't you?* and let her answer for herself.

I'd also like to say a word here about using a person's name. While, as I've noted, it's important, I think residential care communities who are critical of staff who use terms of endearment – sweetie, honey, dear – may be over-reacting. If a garage mechanic calls me "Sweetie," I know he's being condescending, and even though he may be justified in the sense that I *am* an airhead about my car, I'm offended. But many people naturally pepper their conversation with such terms, and they mean them sincerely. My experience is that such people are good-natured, down to earth, and they genuinely like people. To be called "Honey" by them feels good, and I take it as a compliment. It's only offensive if they never learn my real name.

Special considerations for people with additional challenges

Hearing

As people age, their vision and hearing usually deteriorate, and this often creates exacerbated problems in people with Alzheimer's disease. Misunderstandings may be rampant:

> *Three hard-of-hearing men were taking a walk one fine March day when the first said, "Windy, ain't it?" "No," the second man replied, "It's Thursday." "Me, too," said the third, "Let's stop for a soda."*

Being able to understand what's going on around us contributes to our confidence and self-esteem. Yet my friend Betsy Brawley notes in her book *Design Innovations for Aging and Alzheimer's* that a third of people between the ages of 65 and 74 have hearing problems, and almost two-thirds over the age of 85 have trouble hearing. Most of these people do not use hearing aids. Of those that do, many have devices that amplify all sounds, including background noises. That can compound the problem, because people with hearing losses often cannot separate background noises from the conversation they want to hear.

Furthermore, hearing loss isn't just about sounds being too soft, but about sounds being too muffled so that people miss important cues, like beginning and ending consonants. High-pitched sounds – stringed instruments and women's voices, for example – also tend to be lost. Wives have complained for millenniums that their husbands don't listen to them. Some husbands are justifiably accused, but in their defense, they really may not be able to hear what their wives say. And screeching – pitching your voice higher and louder – doesn't help. In this case, Professor Higgins is right, *Why can't a woman be more like a man?* She needs to be if she wants to communicate with the hearing impaired. Lower the pitch of your voices, ladies.

You can also foster improved communication by standing or sitting directly in front of the person with a hearing impairment so she can watch your lips as you speak. Speak slowly and distinctly – no mumbling. Be mindful of windows or light behind you that may create a glare and obscure your face. Peripheral vision becomes impaired with Alzheimer's disease so she may not see you on the side. If you speak from behind the person, she may not hear you at all, or you may startle her.

Be alert to the potential need for moving to a more conducive place for carrying on a conversation. Every human eye is naturally drawn to color and motion. People with Alzheimer's disease find it more difficult than the rest of us to concentrate on one conversation when the TV is blaring, a dog is chasing a cat outside the window or a group of crafters is creating a colorful project nearby.

Other people have hearing aids ill-suited to their needs. Author Carly Hellen tells of one highly aggressive resident in a nursing home whose discomfort was solved by simply removing one hearing aid. Two caused more stimulation than he could bear.

On the opposite side, some people with Alzheimer's disease seem to have acute hearing and be hypersensitive to sounds.

Vision

Betsy also makes a number of points about vision.

- **Older people need two or three times more light to see clearly than most of their young caregivers.** A five-year old child has a pupil whose diameter is 7mm which is more than twice the diameter of a person 65 years old. Combine that fact with the older adult's thickened, aging lens and the result is two-thirds less light reaching the retina by the age of 65. In addition, many older people suffer from glaucoma, cataracts and macular degeneration, conditions that may not even be detected in people with Alzheimer's disease because they cannot verbalize their vision problems.

- **On the other hand, for many older adults, glare is actually painful,** causing eye pain and headaches. Betsy notes, "In many cases where shades are drawn and daylight is kept out, the person's desire is not to block out daylight or be in a semi-dark room, but to ease the discomfort caused by glare." People with AD may not be able to adjust curtains or blinds to a happy medium, so pay attention for them to the passage of light through a window during the course of the day. Also consider using sheer or semi-sheer curtains to filter the light.

- **The eyes of older adults adjust more slowly to changes in light levels.** Not only do older adults need much more light to see clearly, but their eyes adjust slowly from a bright outdoor space to an indoor hallway, or similar changes. It may take as much as 10 minutes for someone who has been outdoors to see clearly again upon coming inside. That means that the first indoor space the person enters, such as a foyer, needs to be as brightly lit as possible and should contain comfortable chairs where people can sit while their eyes adjust.

If for any of these reasons people cannot see you clearly, communication is compromised.

General communication guidelines

There is a long list of general guidelines for communicating with people with Alzheimer's disease, most of which can be used when communicating with almost anyone:

- **Introduce yourself when you come into the person's presence.** If you are a professional caregiver, this is just common courtesy, especially because the person with AD may see multiple caregivers within a day's time. As Alzheimer's disease progresses, introducing yourself is likely to be necessary even if you are the person's spouse or child. You may feel hurt when your loved one can't remember your name, but remember that as AD progresses, people who have it tend to think of themselves as much younger people. They don't recognize their 50-year old daughter or 75-year old husband if they think they are only 30 years old themselves. As Barb in the video *Inside Looking Out* noted, *I know I love this person; I just don't know who the heck he is!* You can introduce yourself without being too obvious by saying something like, *Hi, Mom, it's Ann; I'm here for our regular Wednesday lunch.*

- **Don't quiz or test the person.** My father used to drive me crazy by asking my mother, *What day is it?* She never knew, and it shamed her, because she knew enough to know she ought to know. I knew it didn't really matter.

What mattered is that she felt supported and loved. People with AD lose the ability to spout facts, but they still gush with the full range of human emotions.

- **Slow down and be patient.** Slowing down is probably the most important thing we can do in communicating with someone with Alzheimer's disease. Our rushed movements interfere with good communication as much as rushed directions. When you ask a question, wait for an answer before you ask another – and recognize it may be a long time coming. When you give a direction, give the person time to follow it. And remember just as you can read the body language of someone with AD, he can read yours. If you say, *Don't worry; we have plenty of time,* while you tap your foot and cross your arms, he'll believe the foot tapping, not your words.

- **When giving directions, use short sentences, and take one step at a time.** For example, if you are helping someone dress, you might say, *Here is your blouse. Let's start with this sleeve.*

- **Use the same words if you must repeat a direction.** Because it takes people with dementia time to tune in and take action, if you change the words, they may think it is a new and different request.

- **Don't over-explain.** As Alzheimer's disease progresses, the people who have it usually talk less. We have a tendency to fill in those conversational gaps with detailed explanations, such as why Mrs. Jones' son is late arriving – the traffic is bad, it's raining, etc. That will only make her more anxious or more confused. Silence is perfectly acceptable.

- Remember the pink elephant syndrome and **state things positively.** If I tell you, *Don't think about pink elephants,* the first thing that comes to mind is pink elephants, and it's hard to get them out again. If you say to a person, *Don't go outside,* she will focus on going outside. Therefore, avoid negatives and say what you really want: *Stay inside.*

- **Use concrete words.** It's much easier for someone with Alzheimer's disease to understand, *Your newspaper is on the coffee table,* than *It's over there.*

- **Avoid open-ended questions** directed toward people whose verbal skills have diminished; instead, substitute questions that require only "yes" or "no" or single word or short phrase answers.

- **Limit choices.** It is much easier for a person with Alzheimer's disease (actually for most of us) to choose between two things than an open-ended many. *Would you like to wear your pink flowered dress or your blue dress?* is easier to make a decision about than, *What would you like to wear today?*

- **Use multi-sensory cues.** When letting someone know that it's bath time, showing up with a towel and soap helps get the message across.

- Along these same lines: **Assist the person's participation by providing cues and clues in what you say** (For example: *Oh, look, George; here comes Jill. We saw her last week at the art fair.*) We've all done that for spouses who would otherwise not have a clue who we were greeting; keep doing it.

- **Issue invitations.** Don't say: *Would you like to . . . ?* which can easily be answered in the negative, but rather: *We would be so happy if you would join us . . .* which is harder to resist.

- **Respect the person's right to say "no."** When things aren't working, leave, and come back later.

- **Don't take insults personally.** Brain damage, especially to the frontal lobe, can cause some people to blurt out rude statements without understanding their likely effect.

- **Be aware that everything you say can be interpreted in some other way than what you intended.** The 500 most common words in the English language have over 14,000 definitions. No wonder we get confused. Never automatically assume you've conveyed the meaning you intended.

Judge: You say your arrest was due to a misunderstanding? Prisoner: Yes, your Honor. My wife kept saying she wanted a mink stole for her birthday, so I went out and stole one.

And then there was the person with Alzheimer's disease who passed a sign that said, "Wet Floor," and he did.

Building confidence

You can also be pro-active in nurturing the communication skills of people with Alzheimer's disease. Here are a few suggestions for building confidence:

- **Tap into residual social skills.** Many people with Alzheimer's disease remain adept at playing host, carrying on small talk and displaying common good manners. If that's a strength you notice, use it.

- **Ask for the person's help.** Do more *with* a person, and less *for* a person. If you are assisting a person getting dressed, you might say, *Would you help me by putting your arm through this sleeve?* Then thank her when she does. Give people opportunities to serve: set tables, pass a cookie tray, fold napkins – the possibilities are endless.

- **Let the person with Alzheimer's disease set the pace and scope of the conversation,** whenever possible. Some people with AD have found they are better at asking questions than answering them.

- **Ask about her experiences.** *Did you ever . . . ?* and assume whatever she answers is the truth.

- **Ask his opinion.** This is fail-free. He can never be wrong since we are all entitled to our opinions, even if we don't agree.

- **Ask her advice.** You don't have to take it, but she will appreciate being asked, and sometimes there is great wisdom in the responses you receive.

- **Enjoy each other's sense of humor.** Many people with Alzheimer's disease make their own jokes: A woman who put her sweater on backwards made the excuse that she didn't know whether she was coming or going.

Asking a person with Alzheimer's disease for advice, opinions, or about his life experiences can make good fillers and diversions as you assist with dressing or grooming or other daily tasks, but some people may need to focus all their powers of concentration on that task. In that case, silence between cues may be preferable.

For others, the *effort* of conversation can be exhausting. Do not be afraid to opt for silent camaraderie.

Acknowledge emotions

I wrote at the beginning of this chapter about the futility of arguing with a person with Alzheimer's disease. Here's why it doesn't work: If I have Alzheimer's disease and you tell me all the reasons I need to give up driving, and the ability to drive symbolizes for me the last vestige of my independence, we will never move toward a solution until you affirm my feelings about driving. If you ask me to make a huge sacrifice and fail to acknowledge how large a sacrifice it is for me, I will continue to fight you, no matter how logical your arguments are. Reasoning makes no headway when emotions are involved.

Failure to acknowledge emotions is one of the chief reasons communication breaks down between any two people, in part because we don't always acknowledge our feelings.

In Western cultures, men tend to have trouble admitting fear or hurt; women more often have trouble admitting anger or resentment. But all feelings are legitimate, even when they are not or do not seem to be rational. Our feelings are often based on our life experiences, and my life is not the same as yours.

When we acknowledge the other person's feelings, we are aligning ourselves with them. We're saying in essence, *I recognize this is a serious problem, and I will deal with it conscientiously.* People who feel understood, listen better. Because you understand them, they think you are intelligent and sympathetic, and therefore, you may be worth listening to.

But people with Alzheimer's disease, while they may very well appreciate being understood, are not necessarily ready to listen to reason as their disease progresses. Elizabeth Gaskell once said, *I'll not listen to reason. Reason always means what someone else has to say.* Most of us can empathize with her.

That means we must choose our battles carefully, and always be willing to take the blame for misunderstandings. When possible, use humor to make light of a situation (but never of other people's feelings). And here is perhaps the most important tenet:

The person is not deliberately trying to aggravate you; if he were, he would have a different diagnosis.

Common language patterns in Alzheimer's disease

Keeping in mind the fact that people with Alzheimer's disease remain individuals, and may or may not follow these patterns, here are some common communication changes to watch out for in people with AD:

Early stage patterns

In the early stages, people often have word-finding difficulties. It's the sort of thing that happens to all of us when we say, *It's on the tip of my tongue*, but we simply can't come up with the word we want. Sometimes we forget a name or lose our train of thought as we're speaking. Those things tend to happen more often when we are stressed and literally "have a lot on our mind."

Similar to this are malapropisms. Baseball manager Casey Stengel one day addressed his team by saying, *Now all you fellows line up alphabetically by height.* What was the real message? Who knows? Confusing responses are given by people with Alzheimer's disease regularly and can be more upsetting when they realize others expect answers that they can't give. Barb, on the videotape *Inside Looking Out*, describes how when she tried to explain something and couldn't come up with a word, the woman she was speaking with gave her an impatient motioning gesture, meaning, *Well, come on; out with it!* Barb said she was devastated by that gesture. People with AD are often filled with self-doubt; they don't need their confidence further undermined by our impatience. But the fact that Barb could recount the story shows that people in the early stages of AD are often highly competent in articulating their feelings and carrying on normal conversations.

In this early stage (which can last for years), they are most often "tongue-tied" because we ask them questions about events related to short-term memory that were never recorded in their brains. They are stymied by seemingly simple questions like, *What did you have for lunch?* or *What did you watch on TV last night?*

Middle stage patterns

Mixed-up relationships: By the middle stages, most people with Alzheimer's disease are living in the past (or flit in and out of the present), and they may forget who has been born, who's alive and who has died – even in the same conversation.

Perhaps because they have a hard time hanging onto present reality, people with Alzheimer's disease often mix up names and relationships, saying "mother" when they mean "daughter," for instance. For others, using "mother" for all close relationships may simply be a function of diminished vocabulary. If you are an aide in an adult day center and a woman of 85 asks, *When is my mother coming to get me?* You can usually interpret the question accurately if you say, *Do you mean your daughter Julie? She'll be here by 4:00.*

Another woman I know thinks she is still a child at home. When I asked her to tell me her children's names, she named her sisters, and that, too, happens fairly frequently.

Other people think they are young mothers, and they are unable to recognize their grown children because they are living in a reality in which their children are at least 40-years younger. At other times, they may think their grown children are their contemporaries, their sisters or brothers, or sometimes even their spouses if the son looks like his father or the daughter looks like her mother.

Other people may mistake their care assistants as their children. Since they still think they live at home, you must be one of their children, because why else would you be there helping them?

Generalities as a cover-up: When people with Alzheimer's disease have trouble providing specific answers, they often use bland generalities as a substitute, perhaps because they have found they can seem successful in doing so. For example, I was involved in producing a videotape some years back in which we interviewed a number of residents with Alzheimer's disease in an assisted living community.

We asked Mrs. S what she and her daughter did together. She answered, *We go here and there . . . we go one place to another.*

We asked Col. C what countries he had been to and he answered, *Oh, you name it; I guess I've been there.*

We asked Mrs. G what her mother (whom she believed was close by) liked to cook. She answered, *What I like.* We asked, *What do you like?* and she answered, *Nice food.*

We asked another woman to tell us about a place she lived that we knew was important to her. She said, *Well, we had a nice house. It's on the water. And I had my things made up nicely for walking around and of course, there was all the school business. It was very nice. We lived there twice and it was very, very nice.*

This woman's use of the phrase, "very nice," is what we call a **comfort phrase** for her. It's like a verbal security blanket. She knows this is an acceptable comment that will get her through many situations, and she uses it often.

Closely related to this is the person who gives **"pat" answers** no matter what you ask. Some women with Alzheimer's disease will say, *No thank you, dear, I'm fine,* to anything you ask, when in reality they are cold, hungry or in pain, but find that harder to communicate.

Watch out for residents who use one phrase repeatedly. Be careful that you don't miss real needs that are hidden by their inability to ask for specifics. For instance, it's easy to come up to a person and hold her hand as you greet her. If her hand is cold, you can be pretty sure *she* is cold, no matter what the temperature is, and a sweater or in some situations perhaps cotton gloves, would be appropriate for her.

Comfort phrases and pat answers are different from **repeated questions.** The person who asks you the same question a dozen times in 20 minutes really doesn't remember asking you before – and it's the feeling behind the question that needs answering. A person asking, *When is lunch?* may be hungry. A person asking, *When is my daughter coming?* may be feeling anxious, insecure or even fearful of being abandoned. She needs compassionate reassurance. (See Chapter 9 for more on this topic.)

Non-verbal security blankets: Related to verbal security blankets are objects that enhance confidence. There are many athletes who have a "lucky" shirt or cap. Many people carry something in their purse or pocket for good luck or that is symbolically important in some way. People with Alzheimer's disease often have these, too.

- Men may like to carry a newspaper or jingle coins in their pockets.

- I interviewed one tall man in Arizona who could converse easily when he was standing outdoors, wearing his cowboy hat and looking down at those around him. When he sat down indoors without his hat, his conversational abilities diminished markedly.

- Women may carry a purse or a spoon, a decorative pillow or some other household item that helps them feel grounded to a particular place.

- You may even find that giving a person with Alzheimer's disease something to hold while you are talking with him increases his comfort in talking with you. It helps him feel relaxed and more self-assured. Sometimes that something is as simple as giving him your hand to hold – or holding his.

- Some people carry dolls or stuffed animals and sometimes they believe they are real. At other times, they are probably security blankets. When your world is constantly confusing, it helps to have something sweet to hang onto.

Word finding difficulties increase in this middle stage. Not only do people have more trouble conversing normally, but being asked to come up with a specific word (*What do you call this?* as you point to a watch) may be at least momentarily impossible for them. As a result, they may make-up words, called "neologisms" or "word salad." "Thingamajig" is a widely accepted neologism that can mean almost anything, but a person with Alzheimer's disease may use a descriptive phrase that makes some sense, as in saying "nail-banger" for "hammer."

Other people for whom English was not their first language will begin to **revert to their native language.** One of the theories about the skills that are lost when we have Alzheimer's disease is "first in, last out." That means that the things we learned as infants and toddlers – walking, feeding ourselves, toilet training – are skills we are likely to retain until Alzheimer's disease is quite advanced, as long as we have good care. If English is a person's second language, it is not surprising that he would go back to the language of his birth. It's important then for caregivers to try to learn the meaning of key phrases in that person's language. One more word of caution, however: If a person has begun using made-up words in English, he is also likely to be using made-up words in his native language, so even a translator may not understand everything he says!

Late stage communication

In the late stage of Alzheimer's disease, most people talk very little or not at all, although they will sometimes surprise us. Author Carol Sifton in her book, *Navigating the Alzheimer's Journey*, describes an incident between nurse/consultant Anna Ortigara and a woman named

Louise whose dementia was far advanced. They were "connecting" largely non-verbally in a busy corridor. At one end, a young male employee was trying to flirt with a female care assistant, but she showed no interest. Louise suddenly looked at Anna and said, *Mmm, mmm, mmm, he's sellin' but she ain't buyin'.*

And that brings us to the most important point about people in the late stage of Alzheimer's disease: **They tend to understand much more than they can express.** Never underestimate what a person with Alzheimer's disease understands, even when the person is no longer coherent. As we noted earlier, make sure everything you say in front of someone with AD is something you hope she does understand.

Another interesting aspect of Alzheimer's disease is that **rhythm and cadence remain even when coherency departs,** which brings us to the second most important point: **People with Alzheimer's disease always make sense to themselves.** It's up to us to decipher their messages whether they are expressed through words, tone of voice, body language or behaviors. Many people with Alzheimer's disease simply stop talking in the late stage of Alzheimer's disease, and others rattle on and on, but make no sense if all you listen to is the words. Pick up on the *feelings* of that person as she expresses them by her tone and body language and an occasional word, and you may still be able to carry on the semblance of a conversation. I remember one woman whose jumbled outpouring gave me the impression that she was worried about a friend or relative who was ill. I tried to offer empathy in my tone of voice and a few comforting phrases: *I can see you're concerned. I hope she will be better soon.*

My mother, on the other hand, was a cheerful woman who said almost nothing coherent during the last five years of her life, but on most afternoons about 4:00 p.m. rambled on and on and punctuated these "conversations" with laughter, so it was easy to laugh with her and hope I was on target with my responses: *He was a card* or *That was a good time.*

When a person with Alzheimer's disease no longer talks much, it doesn't mean you should stop trying to converse. On the contrary, people in the late stage of AD need more than ever to be acknowledged, to be called by name and to be made to feel a part of things. If you are at a loss for conversation, talk about the weather: *It's a fine day today* or *Gosh, it's miserable outside today – cold and rainy.* If you are a caregiver in a day or residential care setting, it is especially important to greet the people you pass in the hallway; don't ignore them as if they were just a piece of furniture. For family caregivers, talking about the weather may not occupy much time. Consider reading aloud to them during visits – they are likely to love hearing your voice and it takes the pressure to make conversation off both of you.

Know the individual you are caring for

Dr. William Osler said, *It is more important to know what person the disease has, than what disease the person has.* If you are a family caregiver, chances are good that you know your care receiver well, but you may not connect what you know to making caregiving responsibilities go more smoothly. If you are a professional caregiver you may not think you have time to get to know the individual, but when you do, not only will your caregiving responsibilities go more smoothly, but you will have a richer relationship with the person that is satisfying to both of you.

- Know the person's likes and dislikes, preferences, and preferred routines, and respect them

- Know the person's life story and use what you know in conversation
- Know what brings the person pleasure. For example:
  - Who are the people she likes best?
  - What are two or three places where she is most comfortable?
  - What are three of her preferred foods, songs, outfits, activities?
  - What are three things she invariably finds calming and soothing?
  - What are five things that are guaranteed to make her laugh or smile?
- Be considerate of the person's safety concerns
- Know the person's specific losses due to Alzheimer's disease and other conditions and maximize his remaining strengths

Use this list to build a stronger relationship with the care receiver. Also use it whenever you sense a person is uncomfortable.

Three essential guidelines

The best caregiver on earth cannot prevent a person with Alzheimer's disease from being upset at least occasionally. In general, there are three primary things to do when someone is upset.

Step one: **Affirm the feelings expressed.** To affirm someone's feelings is to *value* him, to say his life matters to you. We do not value people because of what they can do, but because of who they are – always a fellow human being, sometimes a very special one.

You walk into John's room and want to get him up and dressed for breakfast. He insists – either verbally or non-verbally – he wants to sleep in. That is a message of discomfort. Acknowledge it. *I see you're not too anxious to get out of bed today. Are you feeling all right?* Pain, illness or some physiological cause is the first thing we look for when we meet with resistance to our intentions. He says he is not sick, so then we check for fatigue. *Are you still tired? Did you have a restless night?*

Let's assume he answers that he is still tired. Acknowledge his tiredness. *Yes, some days it's tough to get out of bed. Why do you suppose we always get our best sleep just before we're supposed to wake up?*

Step 2: **Solve the problem**. Is there any reason we can't be flexible and let him sleep? Do your reasons correspond to his needs or yours? If he has a doctor's appointment or has to meet his bus for a ride to the day center, then keeping him on schedule may be important, but be careful about rousing him just because you want to get on with your own day.

Many, many needs of people with Alzheimer's disease can be met by providing the basic human essentials: food, drink, comfortable clothing, a cozy bed, shelter, assistance to the bathroom, "work" (activity) that feels useful or that's enjoyable, good hygiene and the affection of kind words and a few hugs and kisses. The trick is in deciphering what is really being asked for. Remember the parent, who, when Susie asked where she came from, gulped and launched into a long explanation of the birds and the bees. When he finished, Susie said, *No, that's not what I meant. Jimmy said he's from St. Louis. Where am I from?*

Step 3: **Refocus his attention.** Step 3 applies especially when Step 2 doesn't work. You've affirmed John's sleepiness, but you can't let him sleep in. Sometimes you can encourage John to get up simply by reminding him of the reason, particularly if he sees it as pleasurable. *I'm sorry I can't let you sleep in, John, but today is your art club meeting at the senior center, so we've got to get moving.* If the reason is not pleasant, find one that is. Open the curtains and say, *Oh, it's a beautiful day out. Come look at the cardinals on the birdfeeder.* Or, *I've made your favorite blueberry muffins for breakfast.* Or better yet, bring a muffin and cup of coffee to his bedside, so that at the very least he has to sit up.

Remember everyone's favorite radio station is WIIFM – "What's In It For Me?" If you know the person well, you know what pleases or intrigues him.

An 85-year old man went in for a check-up with his cardiologist. Two days later, the cardiologist saw the old man walking down the street with a gorgeous, young redhead draped over his arm. The cardiologist called the old man aside, and said, "What's going on?"

The man replied, "Why I'm just taking your advice; get a 'Hot Mama', and be cheerful!"

The cardiologist shook his head and replied, "That's not what I said!" I said, "You've got a heart murmur; be careful!'"

Maybe the old man didn't hear his cardiologist right. Or maybe he just didn't like the advice because there wasn't anything in it for him.

5 —Understanding motivation

*Sometimes I think that the main obstacle to empathy
is our persistent belief that everybody is exactly like us.*
—*John Powell, S.J.*

Many years ago author James Thurber updated several dozen well-known fables. In his version of *The Tortoise and the Hare*, a young tortoise has read the ancient fable, and unable to find any reading which contradicts the outcome of the tortoise winning, he is certain that he, too, can outrun a hare. Thurber rattles on amusingly for another few hundred words, as other animals (such as weasels, dachshunds and squirrels) offer to race the tortoise, but since they haven't beaten a hare, he refuses to waste his time on them. Ultimately the tortoise finds a willing hare, and they mark off a race course of 50 feet. The hare beats the tortoise by 49 feet and 3-1/4 inches. The moral of the story, wrote Thurber, is: *A new broom may sweep clean, but never trust an old saw.*

For many years, the "old saw" was that the person with Alzheimer's disease *is* a problem. The point of this chapter is that the person with Alzheimer's disease *has* a problem. People with Alzheimer's disease and other forms of dementia are doing the best they can with a brain that is deteriorating in ways they cannot control. As their language abilities deteriorate, they communicate through their behavior.

Violence is not a symptom

Years ago it was commonly thought that most people with Alzheimer's disease would eventually become violent. I hope that belief has now long been buried in a landfill where it belongs.

The Chinese tell a story of two laborers who were arguing heatedly in the midst of a crowd. A foreigner, noting the depth of their anger, expressed surprise that no blows were being struck. His Chinese friend explained, *The man who strikes first admits that his ideas have given out.*

The story is an admonition aimed at nations that give up too easily in trying to find non-violent means for solving problems, but in reference to a person with Alzheimer's disease who may become verbally or physically combative, his message is *precisely* that "his ideas have given out." He is trying to communicate with a brain that has deteriorated and robbed him of the vocabulary required to explain his need or want. Lacking that traditional means, lashing out is a way of getting you to stop whatever you're doing and pay attention.

But note that combativeness is born of utter frustration. It is not a normal result of the progression of Alzheimer's disease. Violence may be more common in the person with AD who has a history of alcoholism, or such psychiatric problems as schizophrenia or bipolar disorder. Violence may also be a rare side-effect of a number of drugs, including benzodiazepines (such as Librium, Valium, Xanax, Halcion, Ativan, Dalmane, and Resoril).

Tune in

When we pay careful attention to another person, we say we are "attuned" to the other person's thoughts. "Attune," not surprisingly, has a musical basis; it means "to bring into harmony." As caregivers, it is always our goal to bring our relationship with the care receiver – and that person with his environment – back into harmony, which begins by hearing his song. Remember that *the person with Alzheimer's disease always makes sense to himself.*

  Alzheimer's basic caregiving

I like to compare the person with AD to the cross-eyed shot-putter. He knows what he intends to do, but his aim is a little off, so he keeps the crowd on their toes. Pay attention, and you're not likely to get unexpectedly clobbered.

The big five

Whenever we are confronted with someone who seems anxious, agitated or aggressive, or who is resisting the care we are trying to give, we need to consider "The Big Five".

- **Fatigue.** When we're tired, we are *all* irritable and find it hard to "think straight."

- **Frustration.** When we cannot find the vocabulary to express ourselves clearly or when we can no longer do the tasks we once completed with ease, our natural reaction is frustration. On the other hand, when we have the capability or the desire to do something and our will is thwarted, or people no longer trust our skills, the natural reaction is also frustration.

- **Fear and Confusion.** If we are confused by trying to understand what's expected of us, or if we fear making a mistake or fear for our safety, we will resist that activity or action any way we can.

- **Environmental agitators.** This is such a big topic that I've devoted Chapter 6 to it.

- **Pain, discomfort and other physiological causes.** This is also a huge category. Some physiological causes are easily solvable. Is the person hungry? Provide a snack. Does he need to go to the bathroom? Take him. Is she cold? Bring her a sweater. Are her legs stiff? Help her to take a walk. Others are solvable, but may need more careful examination.

Physiological causes in detail

Because people with Alzheimer's disease, as their condition progresses, have trouble "self-reporting," that is, they can't simply tell you that they haven't had a bowel movement in a week or that they think they are developing cataracts, our responsibility for looking out for their welfare is doubled. In Chapter 3 we discussed the effects of **pain** and **depression**. In Chapter 4 we discussed the effects of **hearing and vision impairments.** Here are some other common causes of discomfort to look for:

- **Effects of medication.** Drugs can have huge benefits, but all older adults need a periodic review and re-evaluation of their medicines, because many signs of discomfort (including anxiety, agitation and aggression) can be attributed to inappropriate drugs, dosages, or combinations of medications, and to side-effects, prolonged use and allergic reactions.

- **Acute illnesses.** We usually notice the person who has a fever, diarrhea or is vomiting, but many people with ear, bladder and urinary tract infections, as just three examples, are only recognized as being irritable or "having a bad day."

- **Chronic illness,** again often accompanied by chronic pain, is also usually expressed by irritability. As noted in Chapter 3, people with conditions such as arthritis are expected to ask for a pain reliever when it is needed; people with Alzheimer's disease can seldom do so.

- **Dehydration** is a common problem among people with AD because they may forget to drink, may not recognize the sensation of thirst, may not know how to pour themselves a glass of water, or may not know how to ask for a drink. People are especially at risk outdoors in hot weather and indoors in cold weather because of the dry heat produced by most furnaces.

- **Constipation.** Not only does its discomfort produce irritability, but impaction can contribute to delusional behavior.

These last two topics are discussed in greater detail in the accompanying book: *Activities of Daily Living– An ADL Guide for Alzheimer's Care.*

The bottom line is that we need to be a constant advocate for people with AD, looking for stressors in all possible forms.

Don't overlook personality

There is a saying: *"Be yourself" is the worst advice you can give some people.* Some people have always been crotchety, and age doesn't change them. A person who has had a life history of intolerance for people of a particular nationality, race or religion may voice this with increasing disinhibition through the progression of the disease. Someone who was shy or modest in youth may be even more withdrawn or easily embarrassed in old age. The more you know about a person, the more sense her reactions to a situation will make.

On the other hand, some people really do experience a personality change with AD. Sometimes they are very anxious and easily upset by the losses they are experiencing early in the disease process, but later, as they forget what they have forgotten, they become more easy-going. When that happens, count your blessings.

Situational discomforts

Graham Stokes suggests in more than one of his books that the discomfort of people with AD may also be triggered by a number of awkward situations. For example:

- **Defensive reaction.** Agitation or aggression may be caused by a perceived intrusion upon personal space.

Often this is related to personal care, when, for example, a caregiver is determined to complete a task such as assisting a person to dress, and the care receiver sees no need to change from his pajamas. The person with AD may also be tired, fearful (not recognizing caregivers) or embarrassed. Related to this is the protection of personal space which may occur in crowded spaces such as dining rooms and elevators or even between roommates.

- **Alarm.** A person may be surprised by someone who approaches unexpectedly from the side or behind, or simply too rapidly. Remember that people with AD usually have a loss of peripheral vision, and are often disoriented to place. In addition, the vision and hearing losses of many older adults can cause them to be easily startled.

- **Competency questions.** Assistance may not be welcomed by people who (realistically or not) deny the suggestion that they are incompetent to perform the task themselves. On the other hand, they may also react strongly when they are frustrated by the realization that they *are* incompetent to perform a task they once did easily, or when they *anticipate* their incompetence, that is, they are afraid they won't be able to do what is expected of them. As one caregiver noted, *If she says, she doesn't want to get out the dishes or make the coffee, I've learned to recognize that she probably knows she can't do it.*

- **Misunderstanding events.** A frail, confused person still living at home, for instance, may perceive a community nurse, even one who visits regularly, as an unwelcome intruder.

- **Reality confrontation.** Typically as AD progresses, the person lives in a past reality. If she believes she must return home before her children arrive from school, she will be understandably upset if you try to tell her she's off the mark by 40 or 50 years. At first she will ask, *Why don't you believe me?* but if you persist in ignoring her feelings, she may become increasingly agitated. Anxiety and agitation are also likely to be provoked if a woman who believes she is a young bride is told that her husband has died.

- **Adaptive paranoia.** I love this term! It is something we all do. We go to the front door and find that our keys are not in the little tray on the entryway table where we habitually leave them. The first thing we say is, *Who took my keys?* We perceive ourselves as reasonable, competent, orderly people, and if our keys are not where they "should" be, it is certainly someone else's fault. It should be no surprise then when someone with AD accuses us of taking his money or wallet or anything else he has misplaced. (The general topic of paranoia is covered in more detail in Chapter 10.)

- **The back-breaking straw.** We have all experienced the wonder of absolutely "losing it" over some minor irritant after handling a dozen far more significant challenges earlier in the day. For people with Alzheimer's disease, every single thing they do requires exhausting concentration, so sometimes an unexpected change in the routine, a forgotten name or a shoe that won't tie properly is enough to cause a surprising outburst.

When your best intentions go awry

You may be the kindest and best intended caregiver alive and still be caught by surprise someday by a person's agitation or aggression. Then follow these guidelines:

- Stay calm in voice and body language.

- Back off. Respect the person's personal space. (While this varies with individuals, during times of distress, five feet is a good estimate.) Often getting a person outdoors is the best way to create "a cushion of air" around someone who is anxious or agitated. The calming effect of regular outdoor activities or walks also act as a preventative measure for many people with dementia who would otherwise be more restless.

- Ask others who are present to withdraw and to refrain from interfering.
- Provide reassurance that the agitated person is safe from harm with you.
- Ask the person what is troubling him. Try to identify the reason(s) for his discomfort.
- Follow the essential guidelines: Listen to complaints; affirm the feelings behind the behavior, try to solve the problem, and divert his attention.

In the future, try to prevent anxiety or outbursts by becoming a detective. Keep asking the following questions until you have detailed answers:

- When did the event occur?
- Where did it occur?
- Who was present?
- What happened immediately before? What was the context of the event?

Then do the same for pleasant events that you *want repeated.*

6 —The role of environment

A real home is more than just a roof over your head
– it's a foundation under your feet.
—Author Unknown

When President Johnson's father was near death in a hospital, he asked his son to bring him back to the part of Texas where he was born, saying, *Lyndon, I want to go home to the hill country. That's the part of the world where people know when you're sick, miss you when you die, and love you while you live.*

Home is where we feel safe, secure, comfortable, loved and valued. It's where we belong. Nevertheless, we are a mobile society; most of us no longer live where we were born, and yet we have usually succeeded in making each new place we've lived a home filled with warm memories and beloved people. We can continue to recreate that comfortable environment for people with Alzheimer's disease whether they are living with us at home or living in long-term care settings, as long as we pay attention to environmental agitators and comforters.

This chapter is about the *physical* aspects of "home." The atmosphere is up to you, and in most homes that's a 50 - 50 proposition. The husband tells the wife what to do, and the wife tells the husband where to go.

Environmental agitators

Two friends, Betsy (Elizabeth C.) Brawley and Mark Warner, are the authors of excellent books on the effect of environment on Alzheimer's disease. Mark has written primarily for the home caregiver and Betsy for the residential care community, but both authors have advice that is good for both families and professionals and that goes beyond the narrow field of dementia. The following advice is taken largely from Betsy's books (See Resources, page 124, Chapters 4 and 6.)

The problems of environment can be largely overcome by creating an atmosphere of warm and loving support, and building in routines that eventually breed familiarity. Those elements lead to comfort. Far too many residential care environments for older adults are:

- Too noisy
- Too poorly lit
- Too inaccessible to the outdoors
- Too difficult to maneuver
- Too crowded or cluttered or conversely,
- Too big, barren, and boring or unfamiliar looking

Recently built assisted living residences were often designed to appeal to the 55-year old daughter looking for an impressive new home for her mother or father. The needs of the 85-year old person actually likely to live there sometimes seem secondary.

Our own homes may contain many built-in comforts, but they, too, may be difficult to maneuver, particularly if a person has a walker or other assistive aid. Many older adults live in homes overrun with a lifetime of accumulated objects that create confusing clutter to the person with AD. Furthermore, noise and inadequate lighting are as likely to be a challenge in our own homes as in residential care communities.

Too noisy

"Too noisy" is at the top of the above list because, along with poor lighting, it causes the most problems. As we noted in Chapter 4, being able to understand what's going on around us contributes to our confidence and self-esteem, but many people with dementia are either frustrated by being unable to hear conversation clearly or made uncomfortable by sounds they find overwhelming. Sounds which do not contribute to a pleasant environment should be reduced or eliminated.

Noise is simply any unwanted sound, according to Betsy. That means air-conditioners, furnaces, refrigerators, outside traffic, running water and vacuum cleaners can all be irritating and interfere with good communication. (One example is landscape maintenance workers who sometimes seem obsessed with their air-blowers. Sweeping is a satisfying repetitive motion, and my guess is many people with Alzheimer's disease would be delighted to help sweep the walks in exchange for freedom from air blowers.) Disembodied voices, such as an overhead pager, also tend to be disconcerting and in this technological age, unnecessary.

Note, however, that even "good" sounds can become noise. Constantly playing background music, for example, tends to cause agitation because it is inescapable. People tend to be less agitated by natural sounds (birds singing, crickets chirping) but these, too, have time-limited appeal. Silence truly is golden for many people, with and without dementia.

While Betsy notes that ceilings, walls, floors, doors, windows, and even light fixtures can be chosen for their acoustical properties, there are many simple ways to reduce noise – especially echoes and reverberations that interfere with understanding speech. Here are a few of Betsy's ideas:

- Carpet floors wherever possible. New technology is such that stains, smells and sanitation are no longer valid excuses for harder surfaces.

The role of environment 79

- Use sheers or other draperies for windows.
- Hang quilts or other fabric "pictures" on walls.
- Upholster furniture or add cushions to help absorb sound. (Specialized fabrics are stain and germ resistant.)
- Hang colorful towels, terrycloth bathrobes, and fabric shower curtains with liners in bathrooms.
- Reroute the television or radio through the stereo monitor for better sound control – or offer lightweight headphones to the listener to keep him from disturbing others.

Lighting also influences communication, since people who are hard of hearing often watch the lips of the person who is speaking for added clues. Some people really do need to see in order to hear.

Lighting

Poor lighting is also a huge contributor to older people's discomfort, and this is as true in people's own homes as it is in residential care settings. **Betsy has six main concerns about lighting** some of which we covered in detail in Chapter 4 on communication:

1. **Raise the level of illumination**. As noted on page 52, older people need two or three times more light to see clearly than most of their young caregivers, even if they don't have additional vision impairments common in older adults such as cataracts or macular degeneration.

2. **Provide consistent, even light levels.** Wall sconces and chandeliers are lovely; however, they can create distracting "hot spots" of light and sometimes indecipherable, even scary, shadows for the person with Alzheimer's disease.

3. **Eliminate glare.** We suggested earlier that people with AD are likely to need assistance in adjusting curtains or blinds and turning lights on or off. Sheer or semi-sheer curtains can filter the light. Glare can also be a problem in unexpected places:
   - Heavily waxed, shiny floors may look wet to an aging eye.
   - A reflection on dinner plates from overhead lighting may interfere with the ability to see one's food clearly.
   - White concrete walking trails may be so bright on a sunny summer day that they cause snow blindness.
4. **Provide access to natural daylight.** This means two things:
   - First and foremost, provide easy access to the outdoors. Betsy is also an expert on integrating outdoor spaces into older adult lives. We both believe that many health and mobility problems could be eliminated if we simply helped people spend more time outdoors.
   - Second, use windows, skylights, greenhouse spaces and atriums to bring outdoor light inside. Most of us are uncomfortable being in windowless rooms. The natural passage of daylight through windows also contributes to maintaining our circadian rhythm (our orientation to day and night).
5. **Provide gradual changes in light levels.** This, too, was covered in Chapter 4: The eyes of older adults take longer to adjust to the changes in light levels going from outside in or inside out. They need brightly lit foyers to mitigate the extreme change in light levels and comfortable chairs to sit on until their eyes adjust.
6. **Provide focused task lighting.** Whether eating, reading, or flower-arranging, older adults need more light for concentrated tasks.

Maneuverability

Maneuverability has to do with two factors: the size of the environment and what's in it. People with mobility problems often have difficulty getting from Point A to Point B. Many people with Alzheimer's disease are surprisingly mobile, but a large environment may be daunting for them as well. People with Alzheimer's disease seem to feel safer and more comfortable in small spaces. Auditoriums are often frightening; normal-size living rooms are more familiar.

However, related to size is what the space contains. Many life-long attendees of a church or temple find a crowded place of worship no longer inviting once they have Alzheimer's disease because there are too many people and the faces are now perceived as unfamiliar. Moreover, the number of people who make a crowd is variable by room-size. A normal-size living room may seem crowded to the person with Alzheimer's disease if it contains four or five people, particularly if he has lived alone with his wife for the last 25 years.

People with Alzheimer's disease also have a damaged sense of propriaception. That means they are unsure of where their body is in space. A person who must maneuver his way to the empty chair on the opposite side of a crowded dining room may show his discomfort by hesitating at the door or even grabbing the door frame. He may say, *I'm not hungry,* and return to his room.

Even if a person's propriaception is relatively intact, he may feel unsafe, that is, in danger of tripping over or bumping into wheel chairs or walkers in confined spaces, especially if his balance is somewhat shaky or his vision compromised.

Environment has a particularly strong effect in dining rooms and bathrooms, but that is discussed more thoroughly in the accompanying book *Activities of Daily Living – an ADL Guide for Alzheimer's Care.*

Change can be upsetting

Related to all this is a change in environment. When people with Alzheimer's disease are moved from their long-time home to a residential care setting or even their adult child's home, we want them to adjust quickly, even when all the messages we are giving them as family caregivers (in actions, body language, tone of voice and impatience) are, *EEIIIYEE, I'm so nervous about this,* or *Oh dear, I feel so guilty.*

There is a Japanese term, *nemawashi,* which means *binding the roots before transplanting the tree.* Gardeners who want to transplant a tree, carefully cut the roots and bind them with rope. Then they wait to see what happens, sometimes for as long as a year. If the tree survives the process, it can be taken to the new site. This does not mean you have to talk about a move for a year before going forward with it, but it does mean preparations should be in place.

Too many spouses of people with Alzheimer's disease are put in nursing homes because their "well" spouse was forced into the decision after a heart attack or other crisis. Taking care of someone with Alzheimer's disease does not have to be a matter of continual crisis management, even though everyone will have an occasional crisis. Like a hurricane, you know Alzheimer's disease is destructive, but you can chart its path with reasonable accuracy. At various points, a person's care needs change.

In recent years, the *options* for care have broadened. Although most of us end up ultimately surprising ourselves, you have a reasonable idea now, if you are a family caregiver, of what you can and cannot handle. Start checking out the options for day care, respite care, hiring an in-home companion, moving to an apartment, moving to an assisted living facility or moving only your spouse there. Look at your area's nursing homes. Plan ahead. If your spouse or parent is in the early stages of the disease, you can talk openly about what to do down the line. Consider it an Advance Directive for Housing. If it's too late for that, check things out on your own or with a friend. Only if you are reasonably comfortable with your decision can you help your loved one become so, too. When you feel good about where (and why) you want to move the tree, you can begin to bind the roots up lovingly.

7—Sleep disturbances

*The amount of sleep required by the average
person is usually thirty minutes more.*
—*Author Unknown*

A wise Irish proverb says, *A good laugh and a long sleep are
the two best cures.* For caregivers, both may be elusive, but
they are worth cultivating. They are also complementary.

I have thought for many years that the best thing
residential care communities and spouses who are caring
for loved ones at home can do to promote a good night's
sleep for themselves and the person with AD is to watch
a videotape of *Tonight Show* reruns with Johnny Carson.
During Carson's 25+ years as host of that late night program,
a generation or two of Americans went to bed with a smile
on their faces, thanks to his monologues, silly skits, goofy
guests and animal antics. And everyone knows a happy
heart is one key ingredient to restful sleep. Or as Charlotte
Bronte put it: *A ruffled mind makes a restless pillow.*

Every creature on earth, as far as scientists can measure,
needs sleep, even those that have no eyelids. Without
adequate sleep we are irritable, forgetful, and have poor
concentration and coordination – or as author and poet
JoJo Jensen wrote, *Without enough sleep, we all become tall
two-year-olds.* That's generally not endearing behavior
for either caregivers or care receivers. So order those
videotapes or DVDs (*The Ultimate Johnny Carson Collection*
or *Heeere's Johnny!*) and try to stay awake until you finish
reading this chapter.

Rule #1: Don't make the ordinary extraordinary

One reason I have always been vehemently opposed to using the term "sundowning" in reference to people with Alzheimer's disease is that it makes them seem bizarre – as if the rest of us don't get tired toward mid- to late afternoon and long for a nap or a snack or more comfortable clothes or a calming walk in a flower garden. If the English were deprived of their afternoon "cuppa" (tea), you would have an entire nation agitated and aggravated.

Nearly everyone "fades" at some point in the afternoon. We may take a nap, give ourselves a boost with coffee or a caffeinated soda, or we work through it until we get a second wind. We are so used to the pattern, we don't even notice it. However, when someone has Alzheimer's disease, there is a tendency to observe every behavior with a skeptical raised eyebrow and label it. As we've noted, over time people with AD tend to become less and less able to articulate feelings of anxiety, uncertainty, fatigue, and fear, so they "act out" those feelings through their behavior. When we fail to see the match between their behavior and their feelings, we make the ordinary extraordinary.

As people age, they tend to have more sleep disturbances. People with Alzheimer's disease also have sleep disturbances, but because they often can't articulate their problems, we call them "night wanderers." When people with AD have trouble sleeping, first look for the cause within the range of common aging sleep issues. Virginia Morris in *How to Care for Aging Parents*, writes that more than 1/3 of people over age 65 have trouble getting to sleep and staying asleep. As we age, we tend to spend less time in deep sleep and wake up more easily during the night. Two common sleep ailments that are usually responsive to treatment are:

- Sleep apnea, a condition which causes throat muscles to relax during sleep and obstruct airflow through the nose and throat, literally causing people to stop breathing as they sleep, sometimes as many as 20 or 30 times an hour. The most obvious symptoms are loud snoring and daytime fatigue.
- Restless legs syndrome, which causes a person's legs to feel fidgety, tingly and eager to move, especially after one lies down or after inactivity such as prolonged sitting.

As noted in greater detail in Chapter 3, another common cause of sleep disturbances is depression.

Many medications commonly taken by older adults have potential sleep-disturbing side effects, including many commonly prescribed decongestants, painkillers, anti-hypertensives, diuretics and anti-depressants.

Furthermore, sleep disturbances can be caused by:

- Stress
- Pain – *I just can't get comfortable,* is a common complaint aggravated by osteoporosis, arthritis and other problems related to bones and joints. Although lying prone is a more balanced distributor of weight, it doesn't eliminate aches and pains. At other times heartburn, stomach aches or headaches are the cause of pain.
- Diet – See heartburn and stomach aches above
- Hormonal changes
- Undiagnosed acute illness such as urinary tract infections
- Inactivity or its opposite, too much activity that leaves us overtired

Since people with Alzheimer's disease cannot express all this, it is up to us to see that they receive the nurturing and medical care they need.

Rule #2: Look for other logical solutions

In 1986, Donna Cohen, Ph.D. and Carl Eisdorfer, Ph.D., M.D., wrote a compassionate book about Alzheimer's disease called *The Loss of Self*. One story from that pioneering guide that has always stayed with me featured a woman named Grace and her husband Ronald who had AD. They had been happily married for 50 years and Grace had always prided herself on meeting Ronald's needs until he started getting up eight or ten times a night, going to the kitchen and holding his pajamas over the stove burners. On several occasions, he ignited them. Once when Grace tried to stop him, he uncharacteristically hit her. This is a classic case of the adage that *All behavior has meaning*. To conserve fuel through the cold winter nights, Grace had turned the thermostat down to 66 degrees. Her wise doctor advised her to raise the temperature, and Ronald slept soundly from then on.

It is well known that circulation to one's extremities deteriorates in many older people, so that they may have cold hands and feet even on a warm day. I once read that many sleep disturbances can be prevented by putting socks on the person as he goes to bed. If he must cross a slippery floor when he gets up during the night to go to the bathroom, it would make sense to use socks with rubberized grippers on the bottom. Otherwise, I can think of no possible harm in trying this potential cure for interrupted sleep.

In that same vein, I have personally found that a light-weight blanket draped across my upper body, particularly my arms and shoulders aids my sleep. I am not conscious of being cold when I don't have that extra shawl-like warmth around me, but I notice I definitely sleep better when it is there. Since my father also always slept with his shoulders draped in a piece of scruffy flannel, I come by this comforting sleep-aid naturally, but I doubt that we are unique in the universe. Like socks on feet, this is a potential sleep-disturbance prevention that seems harmless to try.

Preventing sleep disturbances also begins with other basics like:

- **A comfortable mattress.** Many elderly couples have not gotten a new mattress in many more years than their warranties warranted. Some newly widowed spouses miss the shape of their partner and could benefit from a body pillow beside them. Many assisted living communities provide only inexpensive, narrow twin mattresses to older adults who have long been used to the luxury of queen or king mattresses. (On the other hand, some people feel most comfortable and/or safe falling asleep in a recliner in front of the TV or, in a nursing home, near the nurse's station. Whenever possible, go with the flow, with whatever works.)

- **Familiar surroundings.** If a person with AD moves in with his adult child or into a residential care community, some changes are inevitable, but bringing whatever furniture, bed linens and accessories (photos, mementos) from the person's former home is possible will greatly ease the transition.

- **Neither too much nor too little food.** Most people sleep better if they have had time to digest their evening meal before they retire for the night, but if people eat at 6:00 and go to bed at 10:00 or 11:00, they may be hungry before bed or awake hungry during the night. Some people find a cup of herbal tea or glass of warm milk fills them up and is a sleep aid. Others find the extra liquid increases the number of times they must get up during the night to use the bathroom; therefore, a bowl of cereal or a piece of banana bread suits them better.

Build on strengths

Everything we have said so far would indicate that people with Alzheimer's disease are no different from any of us as we age. To a large degree, I believe that is true. In many situations, their chief challenge is their inability to verbally communicate their feelings and needs.

On the other hand, a mix-up of circadian rhythms in people with AD is commonly reported. People with AD often seem to be awake a great deal at night and to sleep during the day. It's a phase that passes, but it is one of the chief reasons families make the decision to move the person to a residential care setting. Caregivers need to sleep. On the other hand, some of these sleep disturbances may be alleviated with simple measures.

- For years many caregivers were told that daytime napping was a bad thing; now there seems to be consensus that an afternoon nap about halfway through the person's day for about 30 minutes can be beneficial in keeping people from being overtired and over-stimulated. As AD progresses, people usually need to sleep for increasingly longer periods during both day and night.

- Other people may be under-stimulated and require more satisfying ways to be occupied. As noted in Chapter 6, most people with AD, particularly in residential care settings, do not get outdoors on a regular basis. The daily exposure to natural light and outdoor air has a profound effect on our sleep patterns (as well as on our ability to absorb Vitamin D). Others simply need more activity, period. Just as people with AD slowly lose the ability to verbalize pain, they lose the ability to say, *I would enjoy folding towels right now*, (or whatever else might bring them pleasure) and they also lose the ability to initiate that activity.

Whatever the cause of sleep disturbances, we can enhance our ability to overcome resistance to sleep that is not a medical problem by tapping into these known comforters to people with AD:

Set the stage. The atmosphere for a good night's sleep begins much earlier in the day. In addition to getting people outdoors and giving them the opportunity for a refreshing nap, set the tone for a pleasant evening by helping them to participate in a late afternoon activity they enjoy – singing songs, helping with meal preparation or table setting, visiting with family, reading a coffee table book related to a favorite hobby or interest. A bit later, watching a sunset can be both soothing and a natural stage-setter for rest.

Follow a routine. Make a habit of going to bed at about the same time every night. Make the same preparations. For example: Wash hands and face. Get into pajamas. Have a snack while reading a few pages of a book of jokes or poetry or something inspiring. Or listen to music. Brush teeth. Go to the bathroom. Get into bed; get cozy.

Avoid what's upsetting. Don't listen to the evening news, play competitive games or pick an argument with a room-mate. Some people like to relax with a warm bath before bed, but for many people with AD, bathing has become complicated, requiring deep concentration and a fair amount of stress. If a person routinely took an evening bath, it may be better now to start a new habit of simply washing face and hands before bed. For others, the act of changing from day clothes into pajamas is also complex. It might be wise to do that an hour before bedtime, and then do something calming until it's actually time for bed.

Honor individuality. Every book I've read on sleep disturbances says that beds should be used for sleep and sex and nothing else. I have made a habit of reading in bed since I was a child and anyone who keeps me from it in the future will have to fight me. Lillian Carter, President Carter's mother, once said, *I know folks all have a tizzy about it, but I like a little bourbon of an evening. It helps me sleep. I don't much care what they say about it.* Personally, I think she deserved to get what she wanted. (Nevertheless, general wisdom advises against caffeine, alcohol and tobacco before bed.)

Create comfort and safety.

- Pajamas or nightgowns should be loose and smooth on the inside, sheets should be soft, blankets, warm.

- One or more nightlights should clearly guide the way to the bathroom. Shadows can contribute to hallucinations and fear.

- Some people like a cold room with windows open to the night air and lots of blankets; others need a heated room, but like the curtains open so they can see stars and the dawn. Internal thermostats seem to go awry in people with AD; they may be hot or cold at various times during the night and may need assistance with repositioning the blankets they tossed off earlier.

- Noises should be kept to a minimum, and if that is impossible, cover them with white noise or perhaps the sound of crickets chirping or waves lapping the seashore. (In nursing home settings, a UCLA research report found that about 50% of "sleep fragmentation" was due to noise and light changes in the environment attributable to staff.)

- Pay attention to meaningful objects. Some people will sleep best if they can see a picture of their grandchildren on the nightstand, or if they can hold onto a sweater that belonged to their deceased husband (and still smells like him), or if they are covered in a favorite quilt.

- A hand, foot or back massage can be relaxing for some people. Although aromatherapy is still somewhat controversial because of the compromised olfactory sense in people with Alzheimer's disease, many people have reported good effects with lavender-based lotions which penetrate the skin, not just the nose.

Whenever possible, let it be. In a residential care setting, when a person is restless in the middle of the night, there should be someone on duty to be of comfort to that person. Often the cause is readily solvable – assistance to the bathroom, change of an incontinence product, a snack, an extra blanket. If unarticulated thoughts are disturbing the person, the aide should be able to provide calming company, maybe by working on a puzzle, reading aloud or playing dominoes.

In the home setting, the cause may be equally solvable, but the caregiver who must solve it is usually someone who must get up early in the morning, and can ill afford the nighttime interruption. Nevertheless, the better you are at remaining calm and soothing, the more likely it is that the person you are caring for will return to sleep quickly. If you know the person will be safe, you might be able to set him up in a recliner with earphones and his favorite music so that you can go back to sleep. If you can't count on the person being safe, you might have to ask another family member or friend to help or hire a caregiver for a few nights to give you some respite.

Use sleep medications as a last resort and always under a doctor's supervision. Virtually every resource on sleep disturbances warns that sleeping pills should not be taken on a regular basis by anyone. Older adults are especially at increased risk for falls and for unwelcome interactions with other drugs they may be taking. Falls are often associated with drugs that have side-effects of "wooziness," dizziness, imbalance, and next-day drowsiness. Sleeping pills are only one of many medications commonly taken by older adults which may have such side-effects. Furthermore, people with AD, perhaps because of changed chemicals in their brains, do not react in the same way to certain medications that older adults in general do. If you want a sleeping medication for yourself or the person you are caring for, have a thorough discussion with your physician and pharmacist before proceeding.

8 —Mobility, falls and wanting to go home

Take a two-mile walk every morning before breakfast.
—Harry Truman's advice on how to live to be 80

When I was in fifth grade, our school chorus sang a catchy (Swiss?) folk tune, the only words of which I remember are, *Oh, I love to go a-wandering along a mountain path . . . finikuLEE, finikuLAH.* That instance aside, "wandering" tends to have a negative connotation in today's world – to walk aimlessly, even to go astray or become lost. Similar words like "meander" are less negative; meander seems to suggest you are stopping to smell the flowers – that is, the pleasure is in the journey, not the destination, which strikes me as a very good thing.

But the reality is, I am not going to get people to substitute the word "meander" for "wandering" in reference to people with Alzheimer's disease. I am, however, determined to get people to stop saying, "People with Alzheimer's disease tend to wander," as if it is one more example of bizarre behavior, that on the contrary, is completely logical. People with AD walk about for a great many reasons that they may be unable to articulate. It is up to us to decide whether we can "let it be" or need to find a solution. In most instances, we ought to be *celebrating t*he fact that they seem to have a strong will to remain mobile – even if it is sometimes inconvenient for us.

Voting with their feet

Most people are mobile and value their mobility enormously. Being unable to walk is seen as a tragedy. Awhile back we walked to school, to work, to the library and the grocery store. Walking was a natural part of our daily lives. Now most of us drive to all those places, but we still put a high value on walking for exercise, whether we're serious mountain-hikers or occasional mall-walkers.

People with Alzheimer's disease have not lost their love of mobility, but by the middle stages, they may have lost the brain cells that enable them to express where they are going and why. According to psychiatrist Barry Reisberg, as AD progresses, between one-third and one-half of people have a tendency to walk away from home or their caregivers. In these middle stages people also tend to have relatively high rates of anxiety about upcoming events, agitation, sleep disturbances, fear of being left alone, paranoia and general suspiciousness, and delusions (*This isn't my house, You're not my wife, People are stealing things*). If we were feeling all these things, wouldn't we have a desire to escape them by getting up and going?

In addition, here are some other reasonable explanations for moving about:

- looking for the bathroom
- looking for food or drink
- in pain, looking for relief
- looking for a bed to lie down on
- restlessness is a side effect of medication
- trying to escape the noise, tension or pandemonium of a room/person
- trying to escape a task/activity perceived as too difficult
- uncomfortable sitting; need to stretch legs
- searching for familiar faces (friends and relatives who may or may not be living)
- bored or feeling useless
- acting on an old routine such as leaving work for home
- desiring fresh air; may be triggered by outdoor clothing or view

Many of these are easy problems to solve and many are clearly elements of the big five: frustration, fear or confusion, fatigue, physical discomfort and environmental agitators. Affirm feelings, solve what you can, and provide distracting activities, but try not to give up the walk. It's good for both of you!

A similar issue: The person who wants to go home

One of the saddest laments one human being can make to another is, *I want to go home.* When spoken by a person with Alzheimer's disease in a residential or day care setting, it can be the source of enormous guilt for family members. When spoken in the family's own home, it is usually the cause of caregiver confusion, and triggers the response, *But you are home!* As noted in Chapter 4, when the ability to carry on normal conversations diminishes in people with AD, a key phrase can substitute for a huge concept. People with Alzheimer's disease tend to "want to go home" for all the same reasons they walk away from any situation that upsets them.

The most important thing you need to know about any behavior you don't understand is that **a person will always stay where he feels he belongs.** People who want to go home are most often expressing a need to feel safe and secure. Home is where we know we are loved and valued, where we belong. Many people who use the phrase are essentially saying, *I'm uncomfortable; I need some reassurance.*

On the other hand, the cause may be much more mundane. Home is also where we tend to be most comfortable eating, sleeping and going to the bathroom, so the person with Alzheimer's disease may be expressing a need for food, a nap or the chance to relieve himself.

I suspect, however, that most people who say they want to go home are just saying they need to be removed from whatever situation they are in. President Kennedy had a code, "TMBS" for, *Too many blue suits,* which essentially meant, *Get me outa here.* Sometimes a person in a room filled with activity becomes suddenly overwhelmed and needs a little quiet time alone. That may mean going back to her room or for a walk or being provided with some other distraction.

If you know the person well, you may quickly realize the cause of her anxiety. If two people are arguing, a person who says she wants to go home may change her mind as soon as they stop. If there is loud music playing – or even soft music which interferes with her ability to hear others' voices clearly – she may relax as soon as it is shut off. If an activity is too vigorous – exercise or dancing – she may say she wants to go home because she is tired and wants to sit down. If an activity is too challenging, she may express her fear of failure as a desire to go home.

Sometimes a person really is lonely for a home or hometown and family and friends and a way of life that is long gone; then reliving it through reminiscence can be comforting. *Do you mean you want to go back to Chicago, where you grew up? Tell me what it was like there.*

Walking to clear the cobwebs

Walking is "a mindless exercise," that is, we don't have to concentrate on moving our feet forward or on the rules of the game, because there aren't any. For that reason, walking is used by many as a means for either clearing the mind from the congestion of the day or for working through problems. A man was asked on his 50th wedding anniversary for his secret to marital bliss. He said that he and his wife had agreed from the time that they were first married, *If she was*

upset about something, she would tell me off and get it out of her system. If I was upset about something, I would take a walk. So I suppose you could attribute our marital success to the fact that I have lived a predominantly outdoor life.

I know many men, including my own father, who wouldn't have dreamed of walking out on their marriage, but they took a lot of walks to save it. Many men used walking as a coping mechanism for dealing with trouble, and it's my firm belief that many men with Alzheimer's disease are still using it that way.

And while I'm stereotyping people, it's my experience that women are more often walking for a specific purpose. In the same way that men will go for a Sunday drive just to be out driving and women drive to get somewhere – the dry cleaners, the supermarket, school to pick up the kids – women walk with a goal. They may try to leave a residential care home, for instance, to get home before their children (still young in their perceived reality) return from school. Some men living in a past reality may feel the need to go to work.

But both men and women may forget why they set out long before they reach their goal, which is why they have been saddled with the awful label "wanderers." Others have *unacceptable* goals. Some years ago, driving home from work in another Florida town, I pulled over behind two frail old women in wheel chairs, traveling down the middle of the street. One was just managing to push the other by scooting her feet along the pavement. I got out of my car and asked where they were going. "Pittsburgh," they told me. I managed to coax them back to the nursing home a block away, but that brings us to a whole new set of mobility challenges.

When mobility is not perceived as a positive

The nursing home term for people like the two elderly ladies is "at risk for elopement." I cannot say that without smiling. I have this wonderful image in my mind of an aged couple escaping hand-in-hand down a ladder for a late-life honeymoon. Unfortunately, that's not what is meant. A person who gets lost trying to find the bathroom can be easily redirected, but an exit-seeker is a person with a perceived purpose beyond the facility. As I've noted, most people in the mid-stages of Alzheimer's disease are living in a past reality or travel between present and past reality. They see themselves as still having places to go and people to see. However, because their sense of time has become skewed, they can often be redirected by gently asking where they are going and following up with a reasonable response. *Oh, dear, the bus company changed its schedule; I'm afraid you're going to have a long wait. Why don't you and I have a cup of tea in the meantime?*

Other exit seekers are much more emotional, and perceive that they must leave because someone else is dependent on them (their boss, their children returning from school). They are beginning to panic over the thought of not meeting their responsibilities, will not be deterred by a changed bus schedule and will resist if you try to prevent them from leaving. Sometimes letting the person leave and following her at a short distance works best. As soon as she hesitates and looks lost or worried, you can "catch up," speak casually to her, and nonchalantly walk her back. Once she is outside in unfamiliar surroundings, she often loses her train of thought.

When this is not feasible, consultant Mary Lucero suggests people need to be "talked down" from their panic. Affirm their feelings, sympathize with their frustrations.

Ask questions about whatever it is they are so desperate to attend to. If a man is worried about finding his spouse, you may be able to reminisce with him. Ask how long he's been married, how did he and his wife meet? Where did they live? Then see what you can do to provide reassurance that his wife is fine and will be back soon to visit, perhaps by helping him to place a call to her. If his wife has died, and he doesn't remember that fact, look for a creative way to comfort him. Perhaps you can help him to find a picture of her to put in his shirt pocket so that he only has to touch his heart and she will be right there. Perhaps a tape or video recording made by a beloved child or grandchild of his can offer a reassuring substitute for his wife's voice that can be played anytime.

When Cameron Camp, Ph.D. was working in New Orleans, he advised a long-term care community to distract a woman intent on leaving by throwing Mardi Gras beads onto the low branches of nearby trees every afternoon. It worked. Brainstorm with your co-workers; experiment.

Falling down

Frequent fallers are a major concern for staff in residential care settings. Physically and chemically restraining people is, thankfully, no longer an option because it A) is demeaning, B) often causes more problems than it solves (including more severe injuries when people try to break free) and C) is illegal in most circumstances. But in allowing mobility to someone whose balance has deteriorated, we also increase the risk of injury through falls. It's not surprising that the risk increases in people whose vision is deteriorating and who are taking psychotropic drugs. But the risk is also high in those who fail to recognize their limitations as their physical vigor declines, and that applies to many people with Alzheimer's disease.

Falls also occur where furniture is crowded or out of its usual place. (Try moving a foot stool in your living room and just see how many times you trip over it before you adjust to its new location.) As I've noted, the part of the brain that controls our propriaception is damaged in people with Alzheimer's disease, which means they will have a hard time maneuvering around wheel chairs in a dining room or wheel chairs scattered randomly around a nursing station. Be sensitive to anyone who may be struggling and provide assistance as needed.

The goal is "managed risk."

- Falls can be minimized by working with people with Alzheimer's disease to get them accustomed to hand rails, walkers or any other support systems you add to your building or home.

- Also try adding cushioning to their clothing – elbow, knee and wrist pads, a helmet, long sleeves, long pants. Several companies offering assistive devices also make hip protectors that fit unobtrusively into a special form of underwear. These have been remarkably successful in preventing hip fractures.

- Enhance visual cues to make way finding easier.

- Find substitute medications for those that interfere with balance and perception.

- Many people have been able to increase balance and flexibility by taking specially adapted classes in Tai Chi and Yoga.

- Falls can also be decreased by keeping people as mobile as is safely possible – accompanying them on frequent short walks, for example. This also helps them digest food better, breathe more easily, sleep better and decreases restlessness.

Guidelines for guiding people where you want them

As I have indicated, a great deal of walking about is more purposeful than we may realize at first glance, but when people with Alzheimer's disease attempt to go places they are not welcome or where they are not safe, environmental changes may work.

If you are trying to prevent people from leaving through emergency exit doors or lobby doors, your options are limited by fire codes, although you may find the local fire inspector willing to brainstorm with you about creative possibilities for your special needs. (There are also amazing technical devices that can help you keep track of the person in and outside of your home or residential care setting.)

If you are trying to prevent people from entering a resident's room or any other private room that cannot be kept locked, here are some ideas others have tried:

- Signs on doors – One caregiver reported that a red and white "stop" sign didn't work because the person stopped, looked both ways and went on through. However, "Closed," and "Dead End" were effective as long as the person could read with comprehension.
- Paint the door the same color as the surrounding walls so that it simply blends in.
- Paint a large mural on the wall, and the door just becomes part of the scenery.
- Hang full-length mirrors on the door.
- Hide the door completely with curtains or hide half the door with curtains to make it look like a window.
- Put child-proof covers or loose "socks" on doorknobs to reduce the ability to get a firm grip.

- If the door has a bar handle, cover it with a dish towel with its ends sewn together so the towel cannot be removed.
- Lay dark carpet or paint black stripes on the floor before the door; these will be perceived as a hole and usually avoided.
- Create an unusual door handle that requires a two-step process that is counter-intuitive (e.g., a door with two vertical handles which must be pulled in opposite directions to release the latch).
- Hang Velcro strips of plastic "Caution" tape across a doorway (which can then even be left open).
- Hang a velvet rope across the doorway like those used in museums and historical homes to keep people out of certain areas.
- Put in Dutch doors so that residents can look out and kibitz over the upper half of the door, but intruders are kept out in the hall by the lower half-door barrier.

On the other hand, be sure doors to important places – bathrooms, dining rooms – are clearly marked by bright, contrasting colors or flags or awnings. Make the rooms as easy to find and inviting as possible. People tend to most often enter doors at the end of corridors or walkways, so make those the rooms you most want entered. (Indeed, as Alzheimer's disease progresses, people may become stuck at the ends of hallways because they lose the ability to turn around and head back the way they came.)

Remember, too, the quirks of human nature. An astronomer can tell us there are 839,575,428,163 stars in the universe and most of us will not doubt him, but put up a sign that says, "Wet Paint," and we all want to make a personal investigation. Curiosity is a major motivator, so use it to draw people to where you want them to be.

9—Shopping, gathering, rearranging and repeating

A woman may set out to buy a house-dress
and come home with a cocktail suit.
—Janet Wolff

When I first started writing about Alzheimer's disease, this chapter would have been called "Rummaging, hoarding and pillaging" and people with AD would have been called aging pirates. In the many years since then we have grown more sensitive to how people with Alzheimer's disease are portrayed. I personally aspire to becoming more radical as I age, so "pirate" still has more appeal than "shopper." However, "shopping, gathering and rearranging" more accurately describe the behaviors of many people with Alzheimer's disease. They are also a better fit for my general desire to remove the stigma of bizarreness from their actions.

The logic behind the behaviors

People with Alzheimer's disease frequently can be found going through dresser drawers, clothes closets and supply pantries. Their motives may be to find something, rearrange things or hide things. For example:

People who are "**shopping**" may simply like to shop and going through drawers or closets is satisfying that desire, particularly if they are no longer able to actually go to the local mall to check out current sales. As AD progresses, they tend to be looking for anything interesting that catches their eye as opposed to specific things such as a new purse that they may have shopped for earlier. In the later stages of the disease, they no longer have a sense of what belongs to them as opposed to someone else, so anything appealing they see automatically becomes "theirs." In residential care settings, we may inadvertently encourage this by telling them this is their home now; everything in our home is ours, so why should anyone object if we take something?

What used to be called "hoarding" is now called by the gentler term "**gathering**." Many of today's older adults were strongly influenced by their experiences living through the Great Depression of the 1930's; consequently financial security, saving for "a rainy day" and making sure they have "enough" of anything were strong motivators throughout their lives. They may have been people who stuffed their purses with extra crackers and sugar packets from restaurants for years. They may have been people who bought "a pair and a spare" of every important item. They have a real fear of "doing without."

Others gather up items to "keep them safe." Whatever is appealing may be hidden in their dresser drawers or other places so that it will be there when they need it. The problem, of course, is that due to their short-term memory loss, they tend to forget what they have hidden and where they have hidden it almost immediately after they hide it. My mother was a generous person who often had to conceal her generosity from my more frugal father. Once when I cleaned their house after they had gone north for the summer, I found dozens of dollar bills among her pajamas in her bureau drawer. She also had a sweet tooth; another time a drawer contained a large supply of stale candy bars.

Other people spend a great deal of time "**re-arranging**." Some people actually seem to derive pleasure from moving furniture about, and may prove helpful in stacking chairs after a social event, for example, if they are not at risk for injury. Others don't actually move things about as much as "mess up" drawers. In that case they are often looking for a specific belonging that is missing – often something they have hidden for safe-keeping. Sometimes they are simply looking for something familiar or reassuring; this can be a way of "acting out" their sense of loss as their mind deteriorates. Others will take a specific item from one place in order to put it "where it belongs."

What you can do

Sometimes someone in a residential care community will take something belonging to another resident that creates momentary disruption. But often shopping, gathering and rearranging cause little harm and can be ignored or easily redirected.

Here are a few strategies to keep in mind:

- Pay attention to hiding places so that objects can be found when needed.

- Attach large or bright identifiers to objects to make them easier to find; use a large bright key ring for an important key, for example.

- Take away valuables such as precious jewelry to avoid the risk of their loss, and substitute costume jewelry. Promise to be responsible yourself for the safekeeping of such items as dentures and hearing aids.

- Keep the house neat – items are harder to find in clutter.

- Always check the contents of waste baskets and garbage before putting out the trash.

- Put locks or child-safety latches on cupboards and drawers you don't want entered or that present a safety risk.

- Readjust your thinking. If your mother wants to keep the silver in a laundry hamper, is there really any harm in that? The same applies to a residential care setting. If Mrs. Jones puts her knife and fork in her purse after every meal, can you let it be and occasionally trade them out?

Another idea is to create safe, acceptable areas to shop, gather and rearrange. Some assisted living communities have an alcove with a hat rack stacked with vintage hats and a dressing table where the drawers are filled with costume jewelry and fancy gloves. Residents are encouraged to explore the space and take anything that strikes their fancy.

Also pay attention to past occupations and hobbies that might influence these behaviors. One man who moved to a residential care community at first stayed in his room rearranging his socks. He had been an auto parts salesman and had spent a long career retrieving things from bins. To provide him with a more stimulating activity, he was given a set of small drawers filled with miscellaneous non-hazardous auto parts to rearrange to his heart's content. Other men have found pleasure in tool boxes with screws and bolts to sort and tackle boxes with fishing gear to peruse (with hooks removed). Know the person; then use your imagination to find ways to occupy him pleasurably.

Note, too, that shopping, gathering and rearranging in some people may be a sign of boredom. Look for more meaningful ways to engage them.

When an item is not for sale

Jayne Clairmont, owner of English Rose Suites, a series of Alzheimer's specific small group homes in the Minneapolis area, has filled each of the homes with beautiful china cabinets and end tables filled with lovely and fragile knick-knacks. Everywhere are precious objects to admire, but the interesting thing is that most people ignore them, just as we ignore most of the decorative elements in our own homes. They contribute to our sense of place, but we don't feel the need to pick up the beautiful plate we bought in Paris each time we pass it. We can worry too much about the possibility of people with AD touching or taking items we prefer to keep where they are currently placed.

Nevertheless, there are certainly times, particularly in residential care settings, when a person must be persuaded to give up, for example, a vase of flowers or a sweater that belongs to Mrs. Smith.

The key is remembering, as we noted earlier, the radio station WIIFM – What's In It For Me? If I am holding a vase of flowers that you think I may drop, I will not give it up just because you are worried. Instead, you have to find a reason for me to want to give it up. Perhaps you can offer me something more interesting – encourage me to stroke a beautiful, faux fur pillow or offer me a dish of ice cream. You can also tap into my general willingness to be helpful (present in most people with Alzheimer's disease) by picking up another (safer) object and saying, *Would you please hold this for me?* I will have to put down the flowers in order to pick up anything else.

When Mrs. Jones is wearing Mrs. Smith's sweater, the key is usually first to calm Mrs. Smith, since Mrs. Jones is generally perfectly content with her attire. If Mrs. Smith doesn't have dementia, you can usually reason with her – *I will get your sweater back, but please be patient for a few minutes.* If she also has dementia, tune in again to station WIIFM and offer something more appealing to Mrs. Smith. Affirm her feelings, (*I can see you are upset; I would be, too*) and then offer her an alternative until you can retrieve her sweater – perhaps you can wrap her in a luxurious shawl and have her sit on a glider in the garden with another caregiver; use your imagination.

Then return to Mrs. Jones and tune into station WIIFM from *her* viewpoint. What will make her give up the sweater? Perhaps you can also offer her a luxurious shawl or perhaps you can appeal to her vanity: *That sweater doesn't do justice to your pretty eyes; let's try this one on instead*, as you offer her a striking blue alternative. Or: *That sweater doesn't match your blouse; this one works better.* Other people have found success in finding actual flaws in the clothing they are trying to get a person to remove. Carly Hellen tells the story of a man who refused to remove a woman's coat he had taken a liking to until his caregiver pointed out that the sleeves were too short, and she would take the coat to a seamstress for alterations.

Repetitive actions

This topic doesn't actually fit well in any particular chapter, but I've put it here because repetitive actions, like the others in this chapter, are most often a minor problem far more upsetting to caregivers than to the person with Alzheimer's disease. The technical term for repetitive words or actions is perseveration. Many repetitive actions are actually soothing to the person – think of the comfort of a rocking chair or a glider on a porch, or even the satisfaction in knitting or whittling. Walking can be a satisfying repetitive action exercise. **Repetitive actions that are causing no harm can often be ignored.**

People who repeat the same question over and over are also trying to reassure themselves, but are foiled in the attempt. Jitka Zgola, in *Care That Works*, suggests that we do something similar when we look up a phone number in a directory and then repeat it to ourselves over and over until we can transfer it to a pad of paper for easier reading. As soon as we get it written down, chances are we forget it, because now it is in a safe place where we can look it up.

A person who asks, *When's lunch?* may take your answer and repeat it to himself multiple times, but minus that pad of paper where he can look it up, he is likely to soon be distracted, and completely forget that he has just asked the question. When he repeats the question, he doesn't remember the previous asking, but, says Jitka, is simply making a *desperate effort to cope.* "It is evidence of [his] *resolute struggle to keep things in place and preserve a sense of control."* She suggests that providing the information is like throwing the person a life preserver. Your calm answer can relieve his anxiety over what is an underlying fear for his safety and well-being and, if given with a hug, may prolong the time until it's asked again, because sometimes the underlying question is, *Can I count on you to be sure I don't go hungry and am well taken care of?* The hug is part of the answer.

Then again, sometimes the solutions are simple. A person who repeatedly asks *What time is lunch?* may just be saying his stomach is growling. Give him a snack. Similarly, the person who repeatedly asks, *Is it time to go?* may be doing so because he is the direct line of sight of a coat rack that triggers the thought. (Move him to another seat.) Alternatively, he may be indirectly saying, *I'm tired. I've had enough. I want to leave.* In that case, leave, if it's possible, or if it's not, find a couch he can nap on or a quiet corner where he can be undisturbed for awhile.

Sometimes finding an activity that brings comfort to the person can bring a few minutes of peace. As skills diminish, look for elements of a task which may still be comforting. The rhythm of repetitive motions such as sanding wood, winding yarn, sorting coins, wiping counters or snapping beans, can be like soothing music to the body.

Some repetitive motions, especially like sticking one's tongue in and out, may be a side effect of medication and provide a warning that the medication or dosage needs changing.

Early in the disease, many people who exhibit anxious, repetitive behavior can be helped by visual and other aids.

Signs or written messages – *Dinner will be served at 5:30* – may be reassuring as long as the person can understand written words. In a residential care setting, a person who misses his spouse may be comforted by an audio or videotaped message from her or by a note from her kept in his shirt pocket and pulled out as needed.

Sometimes we create our own problems. We want our spouse to share the joy of anticipation we feel over a visit from a beloved daughter, so we say, *Mary is coming to visit tonight,* and all day long we must answer, *When will Mary be here? Should I get ready now?* Learn from your experience. Don't speak before it's necessary.

10 —Illogical beliefs: Hallucinations, delusions and paranoia

I am a kind of paranoid in reverse.
I suspect people of plotting to make me happy.
—J.D. Salinger

In spite of that cheerful thought, most people are uncomfortable with the topics in this chapter. I hope to put you at ease.

Delusions

Delusions are beliefs that remain fixed in a person's mind despite rational evidence to the contrary. Among the examples Lisa Gwyther gave in the 1985 edition of her book, *Care of Alzheimer's Patients: A Manual for Nursing Home Staff* (since updated) are these:

- A 90-year old woman who believed she was pregnant and having labor pains each night;
- A woman who believed she was never fed; and
- An ex-realtor who kept taking the staff's paper and pens.

Some delusions are harmless. The ex-realtor was given her own legal pad and pen, and although she could no longer speak coherently, derived pleasure from writing lists of things to do each day, based on her career. Going along with her delusion supported her sense of self-worth and her pleasant work memories.

Some delusions are primarily family relations problems. The nursing home resident who believed she wasn't being fed, complained to her daughter, who complained to the staff. As their short-term memory deteriorates with the progressive brain damage of Alzheimer's disease, many people forget they have just eaten. The daughter was encouraged to visit at mealtimes to see for herself that her mother was eating well. Many family members bring on this delusion inadvertently by asking questions related to short term memory: *What did you have for lunch, Mom?* When Mom can't remember, she says what seems logical: *I didn't have any lunch.* Of course that upsets the daughter, who complains to staff, and we have the scenario described above.

On the other hand, such delusions should never be dismissed as nonsense, because there is usually a logical basis. Perhaps the woman was hungry. The hypothalamus is the part of the brain related to feelings of hunger. When damage occurs, many people with Alzheimer's disease do not feel satiated even after eating. They may require more frequent, smaller meals at regular intervals or at least regular healthy snacks as meal supplements. Also, people in the late stages may have a strong taste for sweets, but sweets do not "stick to the tummy" like complex carbohydrates and protein. Others may need greater assistance with eating than they are receiving.

Rational explanations do not dissipate delusions since, by definition, a delusion is an irrational thought. Thus, Lisa suggests that the 90-year old woman who thinks she's pregnant and in labor is not going to be convinced otherwise if you tell her such a feat "would make medical history." Nor is it appropriate to pretend to deliver the baby in an attempt to end the delusion. The real message here is that the woman is in physical and/or emotional pain. Affirm that and assure her that you will help her through it. Hold her hand. Might there be a rational cause for her pain? Did whatever she ate for dinner disagree with her? Or is she hungry again? Would warm milk and crackers or herbal tea calm her for the night? Does her stomach get upset because she is frightened by the night – by a strange bed, scary sounds and shadows, an unfamiliar environment? Or is she reliving a past experience? Perhaps there is an unresolved conflict causing this delusion that will need a psychiatrist's attention, but for now soothing words that affirm her feelings and a gentle touch may go a long way.

Remember that people with Alzheimer's disease are trying to make sense, based on past experiences, of a confusing present. Delusions that are upsetting and expressing discomfort are most often a convoluted way of expressing pain. As we have noted several times now, for reasons we don't yet understand, the person with Alzheimer's disease tends to have difficulty being straightforward. If you suspect a person is in pain, relieve the discomfort and the delusion *may* disappear.

On the other hand, delusions can offer clues to potentially valued activities. Women with perceived obligations to their children will likely derive pleasure from intergenerational activities; people for whom a career or particular hobby was the source of great satisfaction will value symbols and activities related to that career or hobby.

Paranoia

Closely related to delusions is paranoia, but whereas delusions tend to be inner-directed (*I have to go to work now,*) paranoia involves blaming others (*Someone stole my money.*) Again it's important to look for the truth in what is being said. It is an unfortunate fact that some unscrupulous people do prey on the vulnerable; the person with Alzheimer's disease who is still living alone or out and about in the public world may indeed have money, credit cards and other valuables stolen. Also as noted in Chapter 9, in a nursing home setting, some people with AD may take whatever is appealing to them from another person's room.

Often, however, the person who blames others does so out of fear. He may sense that something is wrong with his mind; by blaming others, he is distancing himself from the problem. Chances are he hid his money to keep it safe, but because his short-term memory has deteriorated, he has no idea where it is. *Someone stole it*, becomes his cover-up. (As noted in Chapter 5, this is known as "adaptive paranoia.")

Dealing with this sort of paranoia is largely a matter of reassurance. If it's important to find the missing object, say something like, *Oh, dear, I can see that is upsetting for you* (validate feelings); *let me help you look for the money again and see if we can solve this together.* If the missing object isn't important, use the act of looking to lead to a distraction. A search of the book shelf, if the person is someone who has been known to hide money between the covers, may lead you to a favorite photo album or a picture book of old cars, either of which could be a good lead-in to reminiscing.

In some cases, a person may be grieving. Complaining that his dog has been stolen or that he is waiting for his brother to visit, when, in fact, both are dead, may be the person's way of expressing the loss he is feeling. Again, Lisa suggests that you do not have to lie about the reality to affirm those feelings. Saying, *You really miss the dog, don't you? She was such good company,* and then distracting him by suggesting a romp with the neighbor's dog or looking at a coffee table book of show dogs may help the sad feelings pass.

Sometimes, especially as the disease progresses, the source of fear is not losing one's mind, but is caused by an environment that no longer makes sense. As noted in Chapter 6, this is especially true when change is involved. When moving to a nursing home, for instance, it's important

  Alzheimer's basic caregiving

to eliminate every frightening aspect possible (comfortable light and sound levels are key), to bring familiar and beloved furniture and accessories, and to provide multiple cues to help the person find his way. It is often necessary to provide actual physical guidance from place to place, at least temporarily.

Spousal infidelity is perhaps the most difficult accusation for families to deal with. Well spouses have a hard time not over-reacting. Many husbands and wives have devoted themselves so completely to caring for their spouses that they have given up virtually all contact with friends, all of the social life they once valued. Many are too exhausted by these responsibilities to even think about a sex life with or without their spouses. They are deeply hurt by the unjust accusations and the perceived ingratitude. On the other hand, some well spouses do withdraw from intimacy for many legitimate reasons, and the person with Alzheimer's disease may sense this change in the relationship.

Closely tied to accusations of infidelity are fears of abandonment. In this case, well spouses may feel guilty, more often because of their thoughts than actions. No one hopes a difficult time will last forever. On the contrary, we derive hope from the belief that it will pass. To fantasize about escape when you're having a bad day is a normal, and probably healthy, coping mechanism. You've dreamed about having dinner again with someone who can carry on a normal conversation. How pleasant it would be to be held by someone who remembers your name and your relationship! What a treat to imagine cruising to a South Sea island for a vacation!

Recognize, however, that your spouse cannot read your mind. People with Alzheimer's disease who accuse their spouses of infidelity need reassurance to overcome their fears, not scolding for being ridiculous or ungrateful. Join their journey. If you knew your mind was being damaged by Alzheimer's disease, you would probably fear that your spouse or other family members might abandon you, too. If your sense of reality were distorted by AD, you might even think your spouse had fallen in love with someone new. Tell the person that you and others who love them will do all you can to help them through this challenging time.

But again, look for what is triggering the behavior – one woman found that it was the adulterous affair occurring on her favorite soap opera that set off her husband's accusations. As their Alzheimer's disease progresses, people cannot separate what is happening on TV from reality. Watch what you watch!

Hallucinations

Hallucinations are sensory experiences which can't be verified by others. In people with Alzheimer's disease, this most often involves seeing and hearing things that aren't there, but other senses may be involved. One man smelled fresh paint and saw someone painting his living room. Persons who see bugs crawling on their arms often feel them as well. As we noted in Chapter 1, visual and auditory hallucinations are also quite common in people with Dementia with Lewy Bodies.

Like some delusions, some hallucinations are harmless and can be easily ignored. My mother carried on conversations with imaginary companions for years. They kept her occupied and often made her laugh.

Sometimes hallucinations are difficult to distinguish from nightmares, and like them, can be dissipated by spending some time in a well-lighted room where trusted caregivers offer attention and reassurance.

Hallucinations should also be checked out for any element of truth. A person in a nursing home who complains that strangers are entering her room in the night may be frightened by nurses or aides who come to check on her or by a disoriented person with AD who enters her room.

What we call hallucinations may really be simple visual impairment. Lisa Gwyther notes that glare from a window may be perceived as a snowstorm by a person with poor eyesight, who then feels cold. Nighttime landscape lighting can look like fire. Ask the person to point to where he is seeing something, and try to find a logical explanation.

Many people will pick at their hands or clothing perceiving lint or spots, which is generally harmless; often they can be easily distracted by engaging them in an activity. However, persons who perceive bugs crawling on them are likely to scratch themselves and create the potential for infection. Trying to convince them no bugs are there is denying their reality, when they need affirmation – *I know this is scary for you.* Sometimes seeing bugs or worms is a side effect of a fever, infection, or prescription drugs. None of these potential causes should be overlooked.

Medication can also be used to reduce anxiety levels. Check with the person's doctor, however, to determine the best medication and get a prescription. A family caregiver who happens to be taking Valium to calm her nerves might think slipping a few of her pills to her husband is a good idea, when, in fact, Valium is one of several commonly prescribed drugs that can have a negative effect on people with AD.

One final thought: Keep looking for reasons to laugh. *There's an old joke: I've stopped trying to figure out what makes my wife tick. I just try not to get her wound up.* Sometimes that's all you can do.

R esources

This book is based on the advice I provided in my newsletter *Wiser Now*, which was published from 1992 – 1999. My first mentor (and friend) in the field was Mary Lucero who is president of Geriatric Resources, Inc. (800-359-0390, www.geriatric-resources.com). Much of what I wrote in the early years was based on interviewing her about particular topics, and I am forever grateful for her kindness in sharing. Over the years I came to know many experts. I also attended conferences, read journals, others' newsletters and every book I could find on Alzheimer's disease. I cannot provide precise footnotes for how I learned everything I learned, in part because a lot of similar advice can be found in multiple resources, but following are the sources for each chapter that are easily referenced. See also my companion book, *Activities of Daily Living – an ADL Guide for Alzheimer's Care*, for a more complete bibliography of recommended resources.

Chapter 1: Gaining a basic understanding of dementia

You Must Remember This is available from Filmakers Library, 124 East 40th Street, NY, NY 10016. Phone 212-808-4980, fax 212-808-4983. e-mail: info@filmakers.com

Woodrow Wirsig: *I Love You, Too*. New York: M. Evans & Co. © 1990. ISBN 0871316161

A few websites that provide excellent information on dementia and its most common forms: www.alz.org, www.nia.hih.gov/Alzheimers, and www.lewybodydementia.org (There are hundreds more.)

Chapter 2: Patterns of progression in Alzheimer's disease

Barry Reisberg, M.D. is a professor of psychiatry at New York University's School of Medicine and clinical director of the

Silberstein Aging and Dementia Research and Treatment Center there. He has been working in the field of dementia care since 1978 and is author of many books and articles. One place to find a description of his Global Deterioration Scale is on the Alzheimer's Association website (www.alz.org)

Mary Lucero (noted above) was also a primary source for this chapter.

The video *Alzheimer's Disease: Inside Looking Out* by Joanne Frances Durante and the Cleveland Area Chapter of the Alzheimer's Association is distributed by multiple companies including Terra Nova Films, 9848 South Winchester Avenue, Chicago IL 60643. Phone: 800-779-8491 Fax: 773-881-3368. Website: www.terranova. org

Assistive devices are available from many sources, including your local pharmacy, but one good place to look online is the Alzheimer's Store (Phone: 800-752-3238 for a catalog or go to http://www. alzstore.com)

Cameron Camp, director of the Myers Research Institute in Beachwood, Ohio is especially known for his use of Montessori approaches with people with dementia (888 693-7774 or www.myersresearch.org)

Two friends/colleagues are doing remarkable work with people in the end stages of Alzheimer's disease. Joyce Simard is a consultant using a program she calls Namaste (781-588-0876 or). Roseann Kasayka, DA, MT-BC, Vice-President of Dementia Services and Integrative Therapies at UHHS Heather Hill in Chardon, OH, uses a combination of gentle massage, music and "being present." (440-285-4040 or roseann.kasayka@uhhs.com)

Chapter 3: Dementia, depression and pain

Following are the resources used when I originally wrote about this topic in the 1990s:

Jiska Cohen-Mansfield, Ph.D.; Perla Werner, MA; and Marcia S. Marx, Ph.D. *The impact of infection on agitation: Three case studies in the nursing home.* The American Journal of Alzheimer's Care and related Disorders & Research July/August 1994

Betty R. Ferrell and Bruce A. Ferrell. *More Research Needed on Geriatric Pain Management.* Provider July 1990 (pp. 31 - 32)

Andrew A. Guccione; Robert F. Meenan; and Jennifer Anderson. *Arthritis in Nursing Home Residents.* Arthritis and Rheumatism December 1989 (Vol. 32, No. 12, pp. 1546 - 1553)

Keela A. Herr, Ph.D., R.N. CS, and Paula R. Mobily, Ph.D., RN. *Complexities of Pain Assessment in the Elderly.* Journal of Gerontological Nursing (Vol 17; No. 4., 1991, pp. 12 -19)

Ann C. Hurley, RN; Beverly Volicer, Ph.D.; Patricia A. Hanrahan, RN, MS; Susan Houde, RN, MS; and Ladislav Volicer, MD, Ph.D. *Assessment of Discomfort in Advanced Alzheimer Patients.* Research in Nursing and Health, October 1992

Lynn R. Marzinski, RNC, BSN, OCN. *The Tragedy of Dementia: Clinically Assessing Pain in the Confused, Nonverbal Elderly.* Journal of Gerontological Nursing (Vol. 17, No. 6, 1991 pp.25 - 28)

Elizabeth A. Sengstaken, MD and Steven A. King, MD. *The Problems of Pain and Its Detection among Geriatric Nursing Home Residents.* Journal of the American Geriatrics Society. (41:541 - 544, 1993)

Jolene M. Simon, MNEd, RN. *A Multidisciplinary Approach to Chronic Pain.* Rehabilitation Nursing Jan-Feb 89 (pp. 23 -29)

Mark D. Sullivan Mdm Ph.D.; Judith A. Turner, Ph.D.; and Joan Romano, Ph.D. *Chronic Pain in Primary Care.* The Journal of Family Practice (Vol. 32, No. 2, 1991, pp. 193 - 199)

Here are the other named resources for this chapter:

Peter Birkett, M.D. *Psychiatry in the Nursing Home, Assessment, Evaluation, and Intervention.* Binghamton, NY: Haworth Press. © 1991. ISBN 1560240687

Virginia Morris. *How to Care for Aging Parents.* New York: Workman Publishing Company. © 2004 (revised edition) ISBN: 0761134263

Larry Rose. *Show Me the Way to Go Home.* Forest Knolls, CA: Elder Books. © 1996. ISBN 0943873088

Virginia Bell and David Troxel. *The Best Friends Approach to Alzheimer's Care.* Baltimore: Health Professions Press. © 1996. ISBN 1878812351. Virginia and David have written several "Best Friends" volumes since this first one and I recommend them all.

Winifred Gallagher. *The Power of Place.* New York: Harper Perennial. © 1994. ISBN 0060976020

Chapter 4: Communication 101: It's a two-way affair

Albert Mehrabian's work in non-verbal communication is widely known. You can read more at http://en.wikipedia.org/wiki/Albert_Mehrabian

Elizabeth C. Brawley. *Designing for Alzheimer's Disease*. New York: Wiley Brothers. © 1997. ISBN 0-471-13920-3. (See also Chapter 6)

See Chapter 2 for more information on the video *Alzheimer's Disease: Inside Looking Out*

Carol Sifton. *Navigating the Alzheimer's Jorney*. Baltimore: Health Professions Press. © 2004. ISBN 1-932529-04-7. Quote found on page 193.

Chapter 5: Understanding motivation

James Thurber. *Writings and Drawings*. New York: Literary Classics © 1996. ISBN 1-883011-22-1. "Fables for Our Time" also appear in other books of his.

Graham Stokes. *Challenging Behaviour in Dementia: A Person-centred Approach*. Bicester, UK: Speechmark Publishing Ltd. © 2001. ISBN: 0863883974

Chapter 6: The role of environment

Elizabeth C. Brawley. *Designing for Alzheimer's Disease*. New York: Wiley Brothers. © 1997. ISBN 0-471-13920-3

Elizabeth C. Brawley. *Design Innovations for Aging and Alzheimer's*. New York: Wiley Brothers. © 2005. ISBN 0-471-68118-0

Mark Warner. *The Complete Guide to Alzheimer's-Proofing Your Home* (Revised Edition). West Lfayette, IN: Purdue University Press. © 2000. ISBN 1557532206

Chapter 7: Sleep disturbances

Donna Cohen, Ph.D. and Carl Eisdorfer, Ph.D., M.D. *The Loss of Self: A Family Resource for the Care of Alzheimer's Disease and Related Disorders*. New York City: W. W. Norton & Company; © 2002 (revised edition) ISBN 0393323331. The book I used as my reference for this story was the 1986 edition; the anecdote appeared on page 205.

Virginia Morris. *How to Care for Aging Parents.* New York: Workman Publishing Company. © 2004 (revised edition) ISBN: 0761134263

The UCLA study about sleep fragmentation mentioned in this chapter came from a photocopied page of a Nursing Home Research Digest. I have no further information on it.

Chapter 8: Mobility, falls and wanting to go home

Again, I am heavily indebted to Mary Lucero for the original content of this chapter.

I first heard of the hip pads mentioned in this chapter from a representative of Direct Supply (800-634-7328 or www. directsupply.net)

Chapter 9: Shopping, gathering, rearranging and repeating

Carly Hellen. Alzheimer's Disease: *Activity-Focused Care,* 2nd edition. Boston: Butterworth-Heinemann Press © 1998. ISBN 0750699086

Jitka Zgola. Care That Works: *A Relationship Approach to Persons with Dementia.* Baltimore: Johns Hopkins University Press. © 1999. ISBN 0801860261

Chapter 10: Illogical beliefs: Hallucinations, delusion and paranoia

Lisa Gwyther. *Caring for People with Alzheimer's Disease: A Manual for Facility Staff.* A joint publication of the American Health Care Association and the Alzheimer's Association. © 2001. ISBN 0-9705219-3-6. The stories I referenced appeared in the original version published in 1985. This book is out of print.

A bout the author

Kathy Laurenhue, President of Wiser Now, Inc., has a master's degree in instructional technology (developing training) which she began to put to use in the field of elder care issues about 15 years ago after her parents' caregiving needs vastly increased. Her beloved mother died of Alzheimer's disease five years later and it was learning how to support her well-being that prompted much of Kathy's interest in dementia.

In more recent years she has focused on extensions of those original interests: brain aerobics for the stressed mind and life story sharing (learning to connect with one another). She is the author of *Getting to Know the Life Stories of Older Adults: Activities for Building Relationships* published by Health Professions Press (www.healthpropress.com, November 2006) and is currently writing a book tentatively titled *Getting to Know Your Brain*. Other publications are planned on caregiver cheer, creative training techniques and activities for dementia care.

Kathy also gives training seminars (for the public and as train-the-trainer workshops) on brain aerobics for the stressed mind, life story sharing, and sensitivity training for medical offices. She also writes a newsletter and activity ideas for www.activityconnection.com and online courses for www.caretrain.com. She can be reached by writing to Kathy@wisernow.com or calling 800-999-0795 (weekdays 9:00 – 5:00 Eastern time). Her website is www.wisernow. com.

Last, but certainly not least, she is the proud mother of two fabulous daughters and grandmother to two terrific grandchildren.